Instant
Psychopharmacology

Instant
Psychopharmacology

*Up-To-Date Information about
the Most Commonly Prescribed
Drugs for Emotional Health*

SECOND EDITION

Ronald J. Diamond, M.D.

W. W. Norton & Company
New York • London

Copyright © 2002, 1998 by Ronald J. Diamond

Previous edition published as INSTANT PSYCHOPHARMACOLOGY: A Guide for the Nonmedical Mental Health Professional

All rights reserved
Printed in the United States of America
Second Edition

For information about permission
to reproduce selections from this book, write to
Permissions, W. W. Norton & Company, Inc.,
500 Fifth Avenue, New York, NY 10110

Composition by Bytheway Publishing Services
Manufacturing by Haddon Craftsmen
Production manager: Leeann Graham

Library of Congress Cataloging-in-Publication Data

Diamond, Ronald J., 1946–
    Instant psychopharmacology : up-to-date information about the most commonly prescribed drugs for emotional health / Ronald J. Diamond.—2nd ed.
        p.   cm.
    "A Norton professional book."
    Includes bibliographical references and index.
    ISBN 0–393-70391-6 (pbk.)
        1. Psychopharmacology—Handbooks, manuals, etc.   2. Psychotropic drugs—Handbooks, manuals, etc.   3. Mental health personnel— Handbooks, manuals, etc.   I. Title.
    RM315 .D486   2002
    615'.78—dc21   2002070871

W. W. Norton & Company, Inc., 500 Fifth Avenue, New York, N.Y. 10110
www.wwnorton.com

W. W. Norton & Company Ltd., Castle House, 75/76 Wells St., London W1T 3QT

    4   5   6   7   8   9   0

This book is dedicated to my wife, Cherie, chocolatier extraordinaire, who knows more about the chemistry of people than anyone I have ever met.

Contents

Acknowledgments

I want to thank the many people, colleagues, consumers, and students, who have read the first edition of this book and the draft of this edition, and have given me their feedback. Every time I use this book in my teaching, I learn something about how I can say things better. I particularly want to thank my colleagues Pam Valenti and Terri Pellitteri for their many thoughtful comments on drafts of this book. They helped me to keep my values and my language clear.

Preface to the First Edition

This book started as a handout for a series of lectures on psychopharmacology I first gave in 1974 at the Santa Clara Valley Medical Center in California as a beginning psychiatry resident. At that time, nonphysician staff members, from nurses to social workers to psych techs, were not expected to be educated about medications. Though they spent considerable time sharing their experience and knowledge and had much more contact with the patients than did the physicians, they were discouraged from making suggestions about prescriptions and from monitoring the effects of medications. I began to realize that if these members of the treatment team knew what to look for, they could take on an important role in determining what medication might be useful, how well the medication was working, and what side effects were present. These lectures were my way of sharing information with people who had taught me and conveying my realization that medication decisions needed the input of the entire team of people working with the patient.

As patients have taken increasingly active roles in their own care, they have come to be recognized as clients or, more recently, consumers of mental health care. They, too, must be educated as much as possible. By 1987 I was regularly giving the psychopharmacology lectures for nonmedical staff. One of my own clients found the information extremely useful and asked why clients were not invited. My only response was that

I had never thought about it. Since that time, I have invited clients to training sessions I give on psychopharmacology and other topics. At times, this means that state hospital patients leave their inpatient units and go down to the lecture hall. The clients' questions and comments have added to the richness of the teaching, and so far no client has behaved inappropriately during a lecture.

Note that the best way to learn about psychopharmacology is to work with clients—information learned from a book or a lecture can be difficult to remember. The purpose of this book is to give you a sense of the different classes of medications, suggest some basic concepts about medications, and help you build your vocabulary. Your job is to get in the habit of learning about the medications your clients are taking. The way to remember the information in this book is to connect it to a real person. In this, as in many other things, our clients are our best teachers.

Preface to the Second Edition

The pace of change in psychopharmacology is accelerating at what feels to be an ever-increasing rate. Lithium was introduced into psychiatric practice in 1969; although a number of other medications were marketed by pharmaceutical companies, no really new medications were available until 1990 when clozapine and Prozac were introduced. Now, new medications are introduced yearly, all with very different mechanisms of action. In the old days, the medications within a class were very similar to one another. For example, Navane, Prolixin, Haldol, and Stelazine—all traditional antipsychotic medications—all worked the same way, had very similar side effects, and if one did not work the chance of another one working was fairly small. There was little rational reason to use more than one of these medications at a time.

The situation now is very different. While medications within a particular class all have similar mechanisms of action, the differences are much more significant and important than with the older medications. These differences can often be exploited to minimize the impact of side effects. It also means that someone may respond much better to one of these medications than to another, so switching medications within a class makes more sense than it did when only the older medications were available. Finally, because they have somewhat different mechanisms of action and because we know more about what these mechanisms are, we can rationally combine medications to increase their effectiveness.

This means that psychopharmacology has become much more complicated. Getting the maximum benefit from the new medications requires that you understand how the medications work. Medications can often be useful in treating illnesses beyond those that were listed when the medication was first marketed.

The advantage of this extra information is that we have medications that are either much safer and easier to tolerate, such as the new antidepressants, or much safer and much more effective, such as the atypical antipsychotic medications. The older traditional antipsychotic medications had such severe side effects, medications to treat side effects had their own category in the first edition of this book. These side-effect medications are now used less, and so have been relegated to the miscellaneous category of this book and of clinical practice.

More medications are being used by more people, who generally stay on them for longer periods of time. Many physicians are concerned about this trend, and there are books written that are both pro and con on the philosophical implications of the increased use of psychotropic medications. There are also major financial issues in the increasingly widespread use of very expensive medications. A larger part of health-care costs is paying for medications that are more effective, safer, better tolerated, more frequently used, and much more expensive than the medications they replaced.

The world of psychiatric medications is changing rapidly. Hopefully, this book will be a useful guide and introduction to this world.

Abbreviations

qd	once a day	**STAT**	right away
bid	twice a day	**i**	one unit or pill
tid	three times a day	**ii**	two units or pills
qid	four times a day	**iii**	three units or pills
hs	before bed	**c or q**	with
prn	as needed	**s**	without
po	by mouth	**CBC**	complete blood count,
IM	intramuscular		including both red and
	(injection)		white cell count
IV	intravenous		

Introduction

This book is an introduction to psychotropic medications, which are medications used to treat mental illnesses. Medications have become an increasingly important part of the treatment of mental illnesses. Whether you feel that medications are used too much or underused, whether you are a mental health clinician or a client, it is important to learn as much as possible about the uses of medication. This book is for people who are not doctors. It provides practical, easy-to-read information about commonly used psychotropic medications. Although it was originally written for mental health clinicians, clients and their families have found it useful as well.

Chapter 1 provides a list of things to think about before recommending or taking a psychotropic medication. This list includes how to talk with a physician, how to balance benefits and side effects, how to develop "target symptoms" that will allow you to follow how well a medication is working, and how to think about medication as a tool to help you accomplish your goals. I will also introduce you to some important ideas such as "half-life" and "drug-drug interactions" that are important for understanding how to use medications effectively and safely. Medications are most useful when those taking them and the staff with whom they work know as much as possible about what medications can do to help and what problems medications can cause.

Actually, despite the hundreds of different medications, psychopharmacology is less complicated than many people believe. Most medications used to treat mental illnesses fall into one of four categories: (1) antipsychotics, (2) antidepressants, (3) mood stabilizers, and (4) sleeping pills and tranquilizers. By learning something about each of these four categories of medications, and then learning something about a few variations within each category, you will know much of what you need to know. The book discusses each of these categories, the common medications within each category, how they work, what they are used for, and what problems they can cause.

There has been an explosion of new medications. In each category, new medications have replaced the ones that were in common use only a few years ago. The book will discuss these new medications: how they work, how they are different from older medications, what advantages they have, and what problems they can cause.

This book can be read cover to cover as an overview, or you can skip around, reading about a particular medication or class of medications. It is still used to accompany psychopharmacology courses in many schools and mental health centers. However you use it, the book will increase what you know about medications and allow you to use these medications more effectively.

Instant
Psychopharmacology

1

Psychopharmacology:
The Rules of the Game

This book is a distilled and abridged version of my own views on the use of psychotropic medications. Psychotropic medications are used by more and more people for many different kinds of problems. The nonmedical therapist often knows the client better than the physician does and is often in the best position to help determine what medications are helpful. The nonmedical therapist may also be in the best position to evaluate how well a medication works.

Medication is often presented as an alternative to other forms of therapy, leading us to believe we must choose between competing options. The available research suggests just the opposite—that medication, when appropriately used, can facilitate other therapy. Similarly, the appropriate use of psychosocial therapy can facilitate the effectiveness of medication, as well as increase the likelihood that a person will take the medication reliably. This does not mean that medications are effective for everyone or that they are not without risks and problems. It does suggest that all therapists, whether philosophically inclined toward biological treatment or not, need to be as knowledgeable as possible about the potential benefits and limitations of psychotropic medications.

This guide is not meant to be definitive in any sense. Only those classes of medications I believe are most important are covered, and theoretical issues are completely ignored. *The specific indications for use and the specific dosages given are only meant to be rough approximations that fit with my personal experience.* If you are working with a client who is taking a medication with which you are unfamiliar, you can find information about its dosage, contraindications, and side effects in the *Physician's Desk Reference (PDR)* or some other recent medical reference.

While the information in this guide comes primarily from the bibliography at the end of this book, much of it also comes from other papers and books I have read over the years. It is not meant to be an academic treatise, and I have not documented the source for every idea presented.

RULES OF THE GAME

1. *The four major classes of medications.* For most practical purposes, medications are divided into four major classes. These include:

- Antipsychotics
- Antidepressants
- Mood stabilizers
- Antianxiety medications and sleeping pills

These four classes include the vast majority of psychotropic prescriptions, which handle the first-line treatment of almost all common clinical problems. The four major classes cover the most commonly used medications, but I have also included a chapter for miscellaneous medications that do not fit into these major classes.

There are different types of medications within each of the classes. For example, antidepressants include SSRIs (selective serotonin reuptake inhibitors), tricyclics, and MAOIs (monoamine-oxidase inhibitors). Medications of the same class tend to be similar, and medications within the same type are more similar still. While there are many individual medications, each with its own name and characteristics, all you need to know is something about each class of medication and then some details about the major types within each class. If you are familiar with a particular medication, you will already know most of what you need to know about a new or unknown medication of the same type. Learning about a few medications in each class will help you understand the other medications in that class.

2. *Side effects/other actions.* All medications have at least some action in addition to the specific effect you want. For example, in addition to having antipain properties, aspirin decreases the ability of the blood to form clots. Sometimes aspirin is used to decrease blood clotting; other times it is used as a pain reliever. Aspirin taken as a pain reliever has the potential to become life-threatening because of its anti-blood-clotting properties. Since medications have multiple effects, some of which are likely to be negative, you should not use a medication without a good reason.

3. *Drug-drug interactions.* Many medications that are very safe alone can cause problems when taken in combination with another medication. For example, many SSRI antidepressants can interfere with how tricyclic antidepressants are broken down and disposed of by the liver. Giving someone Prozac (an SSRI antidepressant) if he or she is on a stable dose of nortriptyline (a tricyclic antidepressant) can create a dangerous buildup of the latter. Since Prozac stays in the body for a long time, rapidly switching someone from Prozac to nortriptyline can have the same effect if it is not done carefully. Furthermore, administering two different drugs that act on different parts of the serotonin system, such as the MAOI Parnate and the SSRI Zoloft, can cause an extremely dangerous serotonergic syndrome (fever, muscle jerking, confusion, and/or rapid fluctuations of blood pressure and other autonomic systems).

4. *Other medications.* Always ask about *all* other medications the person is taking, including prescription and nonprescription medications and herbal and vitamin supplements. For example, many medications used to control high blood pres-

sure can cause or exacerbate depression. Changing an offend-ing medication may be more effective than psychotherapy or adding another medication. Often people will not mention taking herbal remedies or birth control pills unless they are specifically asked.

5. *Other medical problems.* Ask about any medical problems the person has currently or has had in the past. We are in the business of treating the "whole person," and it is important to realize the extent to which medical illness and nonpsychi-atric medications influence mood and behavior.

6. *Allergic reactions.* Be aware that people can have allergic re-actions to any medication. Ask the client about medication allergies before any medication is prescribed.

7. *Names of medications.* Different medications often have very similar names. For example, Klonopin (clonazepam) is a ben-zodiazepine with anticonvulsant properties. Clonidine (Cata-pres) is an antihypertensive medication often used to help decrease the symptoms of withdrawal from narcotics. Cloz-apine is a new antipsychotic medication, and clomipramine is an antidepressant medication that is effective in obsessive-compulsive disorder. Every medication has a generic, or chemical, name as well as a manufacturer's brand name. A particular medication will always have only one generic name, but if it is made by several pharmaceutical companies, each company will give the medication a different brand name. For example, desipramine is the generic name for a common antidepressant that is marketed by one company un-der the name Norpramin and by another company under the name Pertofrane. The *PDR* lists all of the generic and trade names for all prescription medications.

8. *No one knows everything.* The most important thing to recog-nize is what you do not know and how to get help. At some point, everyone calls someone for help. A nonmedical clinician may get help from a psychiatrist; a psychiatrist may refer to an expert psychopharmacologist. For more information about medications, refer to the resources listed in the bibliography.

THOUGHTS ON THE CLIENT/CLINICIAN/ PSYCHIATRIST RELATIONSHIP

This is a complicated topic that deserves an entire book in itself. The purpose of any medication should be to help the person taking the medication feel better, be more in control of his or her life, and be more functional. Medication is a tool that the person can use in his or her recovery process. This requires that the person be informed about medication issues and be involved in medication decisions. The nonmedical clinician typically spends much more time with the client, knows the client better, and knows more about how the client is functioning and feeling than does the psychiatrist. The more the clinician knows about what to expect from medications, how they might help, and what side effects to look for, the more he or she will be able to help educate and involve the client and make sure that the psychiatrist has the information needed to make an informed decision about medication. Specific target goals for what it is hoped a medication will accomplish cannot be developed in isolation.

The client, clinician, and psychiatrist must operate as a team and, to a large extent, medication decisions should be made jointly by that team. The psychiatrist has ultimate authority over what medication will be prescribed. In most cases, the client has ultimate authority over what medication he or she will decide to take. Next to the client, the nonmedical clinician has the most information about how a medication can be most useful and whether it has worked. Everyone on the team must be aware of the concerns and goals of the other team members. My strong preference is that medication assessments be made with the psychiatrist, nonmedical clinician, and client all participating and sharing information with each other.

It is important to think about when and how much information should be shared. When working with a very anxious, frightened, or confused person who is not processing information well, focus on the information needed to make immediate decisions. Basic information about how the medication might help, ways for both clients and clinicians to determine if the medication is working, and common side effects of the medication should be discussed even with an acutely upset person. Giving too much information all at once to someone who is very upset can overload the person.

Over time, the clinician should initiate a more in-depth discussion of the risks and benefits, long-term side effects, and other issues about the medication so that the client can be an informed collaborator in his or her own treatment. Printed medication information sheets, written at an appropriate reading level, are very useful. All of us absorb less information when we are anxious, and people are very often anxious during psychiatric assessments. Repeating the same information in subsequent visits is often necessary so that people can remember and understand complicated information.

Withholding information about side effects or alternative treatments is paternalistic and disrespectful; moreover, it interferes with the kind of long-term relationship building that promotes effective treatment and helps the client make responsible decisions about his or her medication. Clinicians often fear that too much information about side effects may discourage a person from taking medication. My experience is that a frank, open, balanced discussion that includes a clear explanation of both the risks and benefits can promote long-term medication use. I use my own judgment to decide at first how quickly and how much information I should share, but my assumption is that over time I will provide as much information as possible. Some clinicians worry that clients will stop taking medication if they are given too much information about side effects. If a person is determined to stop taking medication, information on side effects and benefits is unlikely to sway him or her one way or the other. In any case, sharing information in a straightforward manner promotes a healthy relationship that is essential for regular medication use.

Communicating with Physicians

Nonmedical mental health professionals, such as social workers, have learned to communicate very differently than physicians have. Training for social work stresses knowing all aspects of the client's situation. When social workers talk with one another, they illustrate their competence by demonstrating that they know their clients very well. Their clinical descriptions tend to be rich in detail. Physicians, on the other hand, are trained to focus on just the data that is needed to quickly make a decision. When physicians talk with each other about a patient, they present a very tightly organized summary of the patient and the problem and leave out all information that is not directly relevant to the decision at hand. There tends to be little value on information that might allow the physician to understand the person better, unless this would directly help the decision to be made. This communication style is reinforced by the limited amount of time available for physicians to talk with each other.

Nonmedical staff often pass on information at treatment planning meetings or team meetings where there is at least some time set aside to talk about a client. Physicians, whether psychiatrists or not, often find themselves talking about a client in the brief gaps between patient visits, when there are only a few minutes to answer some phone calls or write a note. Time is precious, and the physician has learned to get to the point quickly.

Often, the physician sees the social worker's detailed descriptions as long, rambling, disorganized discussions that never really address the immediate problem. Social workers, on the other hand, often feel that the physician's brief data-based communication style reflects someone who is cold and disinterested or does not really know the client well. This is not an issue of one profession being right and the other wrong, but rather cultural differences in socialization and communication styles.

Understanding these differences can make communication easier. If a social worker wants to communicate effectively with a physician, he or she should try to organize the point being made, leave out extra detail, and be aware of any time limitations. If a physician wants to communicate effectively with a social worker, he or she should use a less abbreviated style and value the richness of detail provided by the social worker.

THOUGHTS FOR THE PERSON WHO IS TAKING MEDICATION

Medication is a tool that may help you cope with mental illness. Modern medications are extremely effective in helping people live with many different kinds of mental illnesses, from anxiety disorders to depression to schizophrenia. Medications do not always work as well as we might hope, and they often have more side effects than we would like. Some people have the goal to take as little medication as possible or to get off medication as soon as possible. I personally feel that a better goal is to figure out how to use medication so that you can have a life as close as possible to the one you would like.

Many clients tell me that they have already tried one or two medications, and that medications do not work for them. They have essentially given up on trying medications, even though their life continues to be very different than they might like, and even though they are bothered by symptoms that get in their way. If medications are tools, and if the first tool does not work, it is important to try as many tools as possible before giving up. If a person has symptoms that might respond to a medication, and if those symptoms are getting in the way of his or her living life, then I encourage the person to try different medications until we find one that does the job.

It is very important for anyone taking medications to get as much information about them as possible. Having this information can help you figure out what else you might want to ask your psychiatrist. It can help you to understand what kinds of side effects you might experience and to be realistic about how medications can help. Finally, having more information can help you make better decisions about whether you are willing to take the medications prescribed by your psychiatrist.

Clients often have questions about medications that they never ask. They find it difficult to ask their psychiatrist questions, or there is not enough time to ask questions, or they feel intimidated, or they do not know how to put their questions into words. It is often helpful to write down questions before the session so that you can remember them. Others find it helpful to practice with a friend or therapist what they want to say to the psychiatrist. Appointments with psychiatrists are often shorter than they should be. It may not be possible to get all questions answered in one visit. People taking medications should think about what questions are most important and which questions can be put off until the next visit.

The following ideas are important if you are going to be involved in decisions about your own medication.

1. *Make sure that you know what medication you are taking.* Ask the psychiatrist or nurse to write down the name of each medication, along with instructions about how you are supposed to take it.
2. *Make sure you know what each medication is supposed to do.* What symptoms is each supposed to help with? How long will it take to know the medication is helping?
3. *Think about how your symptoms are interfering with things you want to do.* Are your symptoms interfering with having friends, getting a job, going shopping, doing chores?
4. *Besides taking medication, what else can you do to control your symptoms?* What have you tried? What has worked and what has not? Often there are lots of things that you can do to control symptoms and achieve your own goals. Medication may be an important part of this, but medication will

work better if it is combined with other ways of controlling symptoms.

5. *Work with your psychiatrist and other clinicians to develop your own list of goals.* Track whether the medication helps you achieve these goals. Are you able to go shopping, or talk to people, or read a book since you began taking the medication? Involve your psychiatrist in your goals. What do you want from your medication?

6. *Make sure that your psychiatrist is aware of any side effects.* Some side effects, like the restlessness that some people get with antipsychotic medications, are extremely difficult to live with. Other side effects, like the sexual problems caused by a number of antipsychotic and antidepressant medications, may be embarrassing to talk about. Your psychiatrist cannot help with these side effects if he or she is unaware of them.

Taking Medication Regularly

Most people with chronic illnesses do not take medications as prescribed by their doctors. This is just as true for people with chronic medical illnesses as it is for people with chronic mental illnesses. This is sometimes addressed as a problem with medication "compliance," but the word "compliance" assumes that the client should comply or blindly follow the prescription of the physician. Ideally, the client-clinician relationship is collaborative, and the goal is to work with the person so that he or she takes the medication in a way that maximizes its effectiveness and minimizes its side effects. This typically means taking medication regularly. Again, this topic deserves an entire book, but here are a few helpful ideas.

1. *Work to understand the person's beliefs about the problem and about medication.* Someone is unlikely to take a medication for a problem that they do not feel is fixable, or if they are convinced that medication is unlikely to be help. These beliefs about problems and treatment influence what kinds

of help any of us would be willing to accept, including what kinds of medication to take.

2. *Simplify the medication-taking routine.* The more different bottles that must be opened and the more different times of day that medication must be taken, the less likely the medication will be taken reliably. People are fairly reliable about taking a medication once a day. It is harder for most people to take medication twice a day, and almost impossible for most people to take medication reliably three or four times a day. Most medications used in psychiatry can be taken once a day, including lithium and antipsychotics. Work with the physician to simplify the medication regimen whenever possible.

3. *Arrange for medication to be taken along with some other regular activity.* Taking medication with breakfast or when brushing one's teeth makes it easier to remember.

4. *Use packaging to help remind the person to take his or her medication.* Plastic containers that allow a week's worth of medication to be divided into compartments labeled by the day of the week can help. At times, I have made arrangements with our local pharmacist to package medication in individual plastic envelopes, one for each time a medication should be taken. For example, a person taking four different medications simply takes the medication in the "Monday morning" envelope on Monday upon waking. This eliminates the need to keep track of pills from several different pill bottles.

5. *Pay attention to side effects.* Take the person's reports of side effects seriously. Even subtle side effects that are unrecognized and untreated can make a person discontinue medication. Akathisia, the motor restlessness that comes from some antipsychotic medications and, on rare occasions, from some antidepressants, is extremely uncomfortable, and people often stop taking medication because of it. Many side effects, including akathisia, can be a problem for the person taking the medication even if they are not visible to others. For exam-

ple, people with akathisia can feel very uncomfortable even if they do not outwardly show the motor restlessness that is a common side effect.

6. *Be interested in the person's medication use.* Ask what medications the person is taking. View changes the person has made in medication use as the beginning of a conversation, rather than as an indication the person has done something wrong. If someone decides to take more or less medication, ask how he or she made that decision. Most client-initiated medication changes are not just accidents or figments of some psychotic process. To be useful, we must understand the client's decision-making process.

7. *Connect the medication in concrete ways to the person's life goals.* If getting a job is what the person wants most, he or she is going to be more willing to take medication if he or she believes that taking the medication really will help get the job. The person is likely to keep taking the medication if he or she does get the job. Continued medication use is often connected to whether clinicians have followed through with promises of assistance that they have made to clients.

8. *Arrange for medication to be supervised when necessary.* A person who is willing to take medication, but regularly forgets to do so, can be helped by regular phone calls, or by visits from a friend or family member, or from a clinician if mobile outreach services are available.

Before Starting Any Medication

1. *First, a diagnosis needs to be made.* Medications should not be given just because a person is upset or because he or she is psychotic. It is necessary first to understand the entire situation. Delirium should be ruled out. Delirium is easily confused with psychosis but can be distinguished by a careful mental status exam. People with delirium are often disoriented and almost always have memory impairment. Medical illness or drug intoxication also needs to be considered, as these may present as psychosis.

2. *Then, obtain a medication history* (what medications the person has taken in the past, in what doses, with what effects). If a person previously has had a good response to a particular medication, it makes sense to restart that same drug.

3. *Pick out specific target symptoms and goals.* Auditory hallucinations might be a target symptom for one person, disorganized thinking for another person, and social withdrawal for yet another. Functional goals are also extremely useful in helping connect medication to real life changes. Monitoring a person's ability to get out of his or her apartment more often, or to read, or to go grocery shopping may be a very useful way of understanding what kind of impact the medication has on the person's life.

4. *Adjust medications according to target symptoms and side effects.*

5. *More is not necessarily better.* Too much of most medications can cause an increase in side effects without necessarily being more effective. Side effects can make the client's clinical symptoms worse; at times side effects are difficult to distinguish from the illness being treated. Too low a dose of medication can prolong discomfort and disability and most medications take days or weeks to work. Some medications need to be increased rapidly because they need to be started low and then raised to get to an effective dose. Other medications can be started at a dose that is typically effective, and increasing them too soon can lead to too much medication being prescribed. These are all issues that should be discussed with the physician.

6. *Actively look for side effects.* Most medications make the client uncomfortable, and all have side effects. Make sure the client knows about possible side effects before starting him or her on a new medication. Actively monitoring and treating side effects will help clients feel more comfortable and will also increase their willingness to continue taking the medications.

7. *Require laboratory monitoring for people taking psychotropic medications.* The laboratory monitoring sections in this

book all indicate what I believe to be the minimal require-
ment for monitoring a relatively young, healthy person
with no complications who is in the community rather than
a hospital. It takes into account the reality that most people
dislike blood tests and that requiring too many will mark-
edly decrease compliance. It also takes into account that we
often work with people who have no insurance and little
money.

Some Thoughts on Side Effects

As already discussed, all medications have side effects. The
side effects mentioned in this and other books are those that
are most common. People are not the same and not all people
respond or react to medications in the same way. Some people
have side effects that are not listed in books or side effects that
the prescribing physician has not heard reported before. All reported side effects should be taken seriously. Some may turn
out to be unrelated to the medication while others may be new
medication-related effects not previously reported. All are part
of the experience of the person taking the medication and need
to be addressed.

If the Medication Does Not Work

The medications used in psychiatry are generally as effective
as the medications used in the rest of the medical world. An
antidepressant is as likely to help someone who is suffering
from major depression as an antibiotic is to help someone with
pneumonia. No medication in any field of medicine works
100% of the time.

As with many of the medications used in physical illness,
psychiatric medications control symptoms, relieve pain, and
preserve function but do not cure the underlying condition.
This can be frustrating, but it is common with most psychiatric
and nonpsychiatric medications.

If the medication does not work, ask the following questions.

1. *Is the diagnosis correct?* Treatment is unlikely to work if the wrong illness is being treated. Correcting someone's biological predisposition to depression is less likely to be effective if the person is overwhelmed by social stresses.
2. *Has a medical illness gone unrecognized?* The most conservative estimate is that 10% of psychiatric patients have unrecognized medical illnesses that are causing or contributing to their mental disorder.
3. *Is substance abuse interfering with the treatment?* All of the common psychiatric symptoms can be caused or made worse by alcohol, stimulants, or other drugs.
4. *Is the person taking the medication?* Estimates are that half of all patients do not take medications as prescribed. A medication is unlikely to work if it is not being taken.
5. *Has the dose been high enough for a long enough period of time?* Almost all of the medications used in psychiatry take days to weeks to be effective. Some medications such as clozapine can take months. Too often people quit taking the medication before it has had a chance to work. Many clients who are "nonresponders" go from one medication to another without giving any of them enough time to see if they would be effective. In other cases, a person will have stayed on a medication long enough but is taking such a low dose that it is unlikely to help.
6. *Are there stresses going on in the person's life that would interfere with the medication?* Medications do not work by themselves. Too often, people with mental illnesses deal with poor housing, poverty, and disrupted social support systems. While medication is important, it is only one part of the treatment process.
7. *Are there other things that the person can do to promote his or her own recovery, in addition to taking the medication?* Almost all people do the best that they can. Illnesses are not their fault. At the same time, if their lives are going to change, they have to be involved in making changes hap-

pen.* What makes symptoms better? What makes them worse? Are there behavioral strategies or activities to help deal with some of the symptoms? A critical part of collaboration is encouraging the client to be an active partner in his or her own treatment.

---

*Adapted from Marsha Linehan. (1993). *Cognitive-Behavioral Treatment of Borderline Personality Disorder.* New York: Guilford.

2

The Basics of Psychopharmacology

BASIC CLASSIFICATION OF PSYCHOTROPIC MEDICATIONS

I. *Antipsychotic Agents* (these are sometimes referred to as neuroleptics or major tranquilizers, but they usually are not the best choice if the goal is tranquilization).

A. Atypical antipsychotics ("Atypical" refers to the class of newer antipsychotic medications that have largely replaced the older traditional drugs. The term is confusing because these "atypical" medications are now the accepted, regular treatment for most people who need antipsychotic medication.)

1. clozapine (Clozaril)
2. risperidone (Risperdal)
3. olanzapine (Zyprexa)
4. quetiapine (Seroquel)
5. ziprasidone (Geodon)
6. iloperidone (not yet available)
7. aripiprazole (not yet available)

B. Traditional neuroleptics (These are rarely used as first-choice medications, except in special situations.)

1. phenothiazines
   a. most sedating; e.g., chlorpromazine (Thorazine)
   b. least sedating; e.g., fluphenazine (Prolixin)
2. butyrophenones; e.g., haloperidol (Haldol)

3. thioxanthenes; e.g., thiothixene (Navane)
4. miscellaneous traditional neuroleptics
   a. molindone (Moban)
   b. loxapine (Loxitane)
5. long-acting injections; e.g., fluphenazine decanoate
   (Prolixin Decanoate) and haloperidol decanoate
   (Haldol Decanoate)

II. *Antidepressants*
   A. Serotonin/norepinephrine antidepressants
      1. selective serotonin and norepinephrine reuptake
         blockers
         a. selective serotonin reuptake inhibitors (SSRIs);
            e.g., fluoxetine (Prozac) and sertraline (Zoloft)
         b. selective serotonin and noradrenergic reuptake
            blockers; e.g., venlafaxine (Effexor)
         c. selective noradrenergic reuptake blockers;
            reboxetine (not available in the US)
      2. alpha 2 antagonist; e.g., mirtazapine (Remeron)
      3. serotonin 2a receptor blockers; e.g., nefazadone
         (Serzone) and trazadone (Deseryl)
   B. Norepinephrine and dopamine reuptake blockers; e.g.,
      bupropion (Wellbutrin)
   C. Tricyclic antidepressants
      1. norepinephrine reuptake blockade; e.g., desipramine
         (Norpramin) and amitriptyline (Elavil)
      2. serotonin reuptake blockade; e.g., Clomipramine
         (Anafranil)
   D. Monoamine oxidase inhibitors (MAOIs); e.g.,
      phenelzine (Nardil) and tranylcypromine (Parnate)

III. *Mood Stabilizers*
   A. Lithium (Eskalith, Lithane)
   B. Anticonvulsants
      1. carbamazepine (Tegretol)
      2. oxcarbazepine (Trileptal) (active metabolite of
         carbamazepine with fewer side effects)

3. valproic acid (Depakote)
4. miscellaneous "new-generation" anticonvulsants; e.g., lamotrigine (Lamactil), gabapentin (Neurontin), topiramate (Topamax)

IV. *Antianxiety Medications and Sleeping Pills*
  A. Antianxiety
    1. benzodiazepines; e.g., diazepam (Valium) and alprazolam (Xanax)
    2. buspirone (BuSpar), a new anxiolytic that is unique because it is supposed to be nonsedating and nonaddictive (serotonin$_{1A}$ augmenting agent)
    3. meprobamate (Equanil, Miltown), barbiturates, and other older medications
  B. Sleeping pills
    1. zolpidem (Ambien) and zaleplon (Sonata) are new nonbenzodiazepine sleeping pills
    2. benzodiazepines; e.g., temazepam (Restoril)
    3. trazodone (a sedative antidepressant)
    4. sedative antihistamines; e.g., diphenhydramine (Benadryl)
    5. chloral hydrate

V. *Miscellaneous*
  A. Beta-blockers; e.g., propranolol (Inderal)
  B. Stimulants; e.g., modafinil (Provigil), methylphenidate (Ritalin), and amphetamines (Dexadrine)
  C. Medications to decrease alcohol abuse
    1. disulfiram (Antabuse)
    2. naltrexone (ReVia)
  D. Antiparkinson medications (to decrease extrapyramidal side effects)
    1. anticholinergic; e.g., benztropine (Cogentin), diphenhydramine (Benadryl)
    2. dopaminergic; e.g., amantadine (Symmetrel)
  E. Cognitive enhancers (for use in dementia)
    1. cholinergic medications; e.g., donepezil (Aricept)

HOW DO MEDICATIONS WORK?

Most psychotropic drugs affect the activity of the brain by increasing or decreasing the activity of various *neurotransmitters*, chemical messengers that operate between adjacent nerve cells. The space between two nerve cells is called a synapse. Neurotransmitters are released from a nerve cell into the synapse. The neurotransmitter travels across the synapse to act on the receptors of the next nerve cell.

Some neurotransmitters are excitatory and trigger the firing of the nerve cell. Other neurotransmitters are inhibitory and inhibit the firing of the cell. Receptors can be either presynaptic or postsynaptic. Presynaptic receptors are on the nerve cell that releases the neurotransmitter and acts as a brake or feedback mechanism controlling the amount of the neurotransmitter released. Postsynaptic receptors are on the other side of the synapse. Different medications work by being either exitatory or inhibitory, either at the presynaptic or postsynaptic receptors, or in a somewhat complicated combination of these.

Each neurotransmitter operates in multiple places in the brain, causing many different effects. More than 20 neurotransmitters have been identified. The important ones in psychopharmacology are *acetylcholine, dopamine, adrenalin* (or *epinephrine*), *noradrenalin* (or *norepinephrine*), *serotonin,* and *GABA.* A number of new neurotransmitters are beginning to be discussed in the literature and medications are currently being developed that effect glutamate, nicotine, substance P, and many others.

Generally speaking, a particular kind of nerve cell will release only one kind of neurotransmitter. A serotonin cell will release only serotonin, and a dopamine cell will release only dopamine. Each cell will have receptors for many different types of a neurotransmitter. A single nerve cell may have receptors for dopamine, serotonin, glutamate, acetylcholine, and more. Even more complicated, each neurotransmitter affects a number of different receptors. There are at least five different dopamine receptors (labeled D_1, D_2, and so on). There are at least 15 different serotonin receptors, with more being discovered all the time. Each of these different receptors has different actions in the brain and different responses to medications.

Acetylcholine. This is a neurotransmitter widely present throughout the body. Acetylcholine receptors are called cholinergic receptors (choline = cholinergic), and medications that block the action of acetylcholine by blocking receptors are called anticholinergic. The cholinergic system controls such things as salivation, gut motility, and the lens in the eye. Therefore, medications that block the cholinergic system typically cause dry mouth, blurred vision, and constipation. Anticholinergic medications can also cause memory problems, confusion, and delirium. Medications that increase acetylcholine in the brain are "cognitive enhancers" and are being used for the symptomatic treatment of dementia.

Dopamine/dopaminergic. This is a neurotransmitter found in the brain. A number of different dopamine receptors now have been identified. Traditional antipsychotic medications block the action of dopamine at the receptor sites in the receiving cells. Specifically, they block what are called D_2 receptors. Blocking D_2 receptors in the mesolimbic part of the brain is responsible for the antipsychotic properties of these medications. Blocking dopamine receptors in other parts of the brain causes many of the side effects of these medications. The "atypical" antipsychotic medications are much more selective and tend to block just the receptors needed to treat symptoms while having lesser effects on other receptors.

Epinephrine (adrenaline). There are two kinds of adrenergic receptors: alpha and beta. Beta-blockers (propranolol) block the beta set of these receptors, leaving the alpha set intact.

GABA (gamma-aminobutyric acid). This inhibits or decreases the activity of nerve cells. Antianxiety medications such as Valium increase GABA activity.

Norepinephrine (noradrenalin). Norepinephrine seems involved in depression and the ability to have positive feelings. Most antidepressants affect either norepinephrine or serotonin in complicated ways. It was once believed that antidepressants blocked the deactivation of these neurotransmitters, effectively increasing the amount available. This view is too simple and probably inaccurate.

Serotonin (abbreviated 5-HT for 5-hydroxytryptamine). Serotonin is involved in depression, psychosis, and obsessive-compulsive disorder. An increasing number of newer medications target different parts of this very complicated neurotransmitter system. There are now some 15 known types of serotonin receptors grouped into five distinct families.

A Discussion about Time

Everything, including modern medicine, takes time, and people often give up on medications or physicians change doses before the medication has had time to stabilize. Understanding the time a medication needs to take effect is an important part of developing a successful treatment plan. Often, the decision to use one medication rather than another is influenced by how quickly the medication works or how long or short a period of time it stays in the person's body. There are four things to consider when asking how long it will take a medication to work: (1) how long it takes for the medication to be absorbed within the stomach, (2) how long it takes to build up an effective level in the blood, (3) how long it takes to get from the blood into the brain, and (4) how long it takes to work once it is in the brain.

Absorption

A medication takes time to enter the bloodstream. An intravenous injection shows up in the blood immediately, while a pill taken on a full stomach may take an hour or more. Some medications are absorbed more rapidly than others. While the absorption time may influence how long it takes for a medication to work, more often other variables have much more impact. How much of the medication is absorbed does matter however. For example, while most medications are absorbed more rapidly on an empty stomach, ziprasidone (Geodon) is better absorbed if there is food in your stomach.

Half-life

When a person takes the first dose of a new medication, the serum level goes up as the medication is absorbed and then falls as the medication is broken apart (metabolized) or gotten rid of (excreted). If a person takes a second dose of the medication before all of the previous dose has left the body, the second dose will add to the remaining part of the first dose. Most medications are eliminated slowly enough that the serum level continues to increase over time, even if the client takes the same dose of medication every day. The ups and downs eventually level off at what is called a "steady state serum level." If the person then stops taking the medication, the serum level of the medication will fall over time.

Half-life refers to how long it will take for half of the medication to leave the person's body. If a medication's half-life is 12 hours, half of the amount taken will be out of the body at the end of 12 hours; half of the remaining amount (75% of the original dose) will be out after 24 hours; and half of that (87.5% of the original dose) will be out after 36 hours. It takes approximately five half-lives for a medication that is taken regularly to reach steady state. If a medication has a half-life of 24 to 100 hours (such as Dalmane), and is taken every night as a sleeping pill, the serum level of the medication will continue to increase every day for 5 to 20 days before steady state is reached. If a medication has a 10- to 20-day half-life (such as fluphenazine decanoate), and is given on a regular basis, the serum level of that medication will continue to increase over 50 to 100 days.

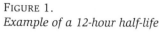

FIGURE 1.
Example of a 12-hour half-life

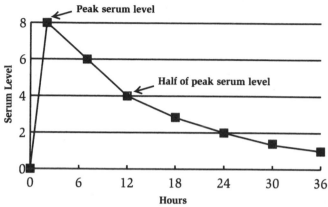

Crossing the "Blood-Brain Barrier"

Even after a medication is in the blood, it may take some time to cross the "blood-brain barrier" and enter the brain where it can take effect. The brain is surrounded by a set of interlocking cells that form a barrier. These cells are highly modified fat cells, and medications that dissolve in fat cross this barrier more rapidly than medications that only dissolve in water. Valium, for example, enters the brain very rapidly, while a similar medication like Serax that is less fat soluble may take longer. Large molecules that are not fat soluble may not enter the brain at all while very small molecules like lithium may cross the barrier almost immediately.

Time to Take Effect

Even after there is an effective serum level and even after the medication has crossed from the blood to the brain, it takes time for most psychotropic medications to work. We are learning that most psychotropic medications work by influencing the amount of specific proteins or enzymes that a specific nerve cell makes. It takes up to several weeks for most antidepressants to take effect, while side effects often begin almost immediately. If someone taking a medication does not understand this, he or she may become frustrated by the lack of improvement, feel that the medication is making things worse rather than better, and discontinue the medication shortly after starting it. Similarly, a person who is psychotic is often started on a moderate dose of an antipsychotic medication, but if he or she does not improve within a few days, the dose is often increased. The dose of antipsychotic medication may be increased several times during the first week. Often, when the person then begins to respond to this higher dose, it is often mistakenly assumed that he or she needs the higher dose. While that may be true, it is just as likely that the client simply needed time to respond and may have responded whether or not the dose was raised.

The opposite occurs when someone stops or decreases the dose of a medication. The serum level may drop in hours or days, but it may take weeks or even months for the person to get the full impact of the change. For example, many people with schizophrenia will not immediately become more symptomatic if they stop taking their antipsychotic medication, but they will be at a much higher risk for relapse over the next few weeks or months. In most cases, especially when a medication has been taken for a long time, one should wait weeks to months after decreasing the dose before making the next decrease. A very slow taper decreases the risk of relapse and gives the person the chance to see the effect of one decrease before making another.

DRUG-DRUG INTERACTIONS

There is increasing understanding of how one medication can affect other medications. In some cases, one medication can increase the effectiveness of another. For example, lithium sometimes is used to increase the effectiveness of an antidepressant. Similarly, one medication can increase the side effects of another. For example, antihistamines like diphenhydramine (Benadryl) can increase the tiredness, dry mouth, and constipation caused by tricyclic antidepressants like amitriptyline (Elavil).

Much recent interest has focused on how one drug can either increase or decrease how rapidly another medication is broken apart and deactivated by the body. For example, carbamazepine (Tegretol) *induces* (increases the activity of) the liver enzyme that metabolizes many other medications, including antipsychotic medications. As a result, if a person already taking an antipsychotic medication starts taking carbamazepine, his or her antipsychotic serum level will go down. Women taking oral contraceptives and carbamazepine are at greater risk for an unexpected pregnancy, because carbamazepine lowers the hormone level established by the oral contraceptives. Cigarette smoking induces the enzymes responsible for the metabolism of many antipsychotic medications, including clozapine and olanzapine, which in turn decreases the serum level of these medications.

On the other hand, fluoxetine (Prozac) interferes with the metabolism (and therefore raises serum levels) of many medications, including amitriptyline and diazepam (Valium). If not carefully monitored, a person taking fluoxetine along with a traditional antidepressant like amitriptyline (Elavil) can rapidly develop a dangerously high serum level of the traditional antidepressant. Fluoxetine has a very long half-life (7–9 days, including its active metabolite) so a significant amount of the medication can stay in a person's body for several weeks. When someone switches from fluoxetine to another antidepressant, the fluoxetine remaining after the switch can cause a rapid, potentially dangerous buildup of the new medication, unless there is a medication-free period of several weeks or the new medication is started at an extremely low dose.

While some of these interactions are relatively inconsequential, some may be life-threatening. For example, the antihistamine terfenadine (Seldane) was taken off the market because of its life-threatening interactions. It was very safe when used alone but could cause a life-threatening arrhythmia (irregular heartbeat) when taken with fluoxetine (Prozac) or a number of other antidepressants that interfered with terfenadine's metabolism. Many of the most important drug-drug interactions center around the newer antidepressants and they will be discussed in more detail within that section. Drug-drug interactions affect many different medications, however, and it is one of the areas of psychopharmacology that is most complicated and is changing most rapidly.

Call a pharmacy if you have a question about possible drug-drug interactions. Most pharmacies have constantly updated references and computer programs that can be used to check the interactions between the various medications a person may be taking. Most pharmacies are glad to look up drug interactions even if the person is not receiving all of his or her medication from that pharmacy.

Drug-Drug Interactions and the P450 Enzyme System

The CYP450 enzymes are a collection of enzymes found in the liver that break down and deactivate a large number of substances, including medications and some foods. They are described by a number followed by a letter followed by another number, for example, 1A2 and 2D6. The first number refers to the gene family, the number refers to the gene subfamily, and the last number refers to the specific gene number. The mechanisms of these enzymes are still being worked out, and only a few seem relevant to medications commonly used in psychiatry.

A particular medication can induce (increase the activity of) an enzyme, or inhibit (decrease the activity of) an enzyme. A substrate is any medication or any other substance broken apart by a particular enzyme. (Note that Table 1 does not cover all possible interactions.)

TABLE 1. Examples of Medications that Inhibit Specific P450 Enzyme Systems Required for the Metabolism of Other Medications

CYP 1A	CYP 2C	CYP 2D6	CYP 3A3/4/5
cimetidine	fluvoxamine	chlorpheniramine	HIV protease inhibitors
fluvoxamine	fluoxetine	cimetidine	cimetidine
		clomipramine	erythromycin
		fluoxetine	fluoxetine
		methadone	fluvoxamine
		paroxetine	grapefruit juice
			nefazodone

Examples of Medications that Induce Specific P450 Enzyme Systems Required for the Metabolism of Other Medications

CYP 1A	CYP 2C	CYP 2D6	CYP 3A3/4/5
tobacco			carbamazepine
			St John's Wort

Examples of Medications Metabolized by Specific Enzyme Systems (and would have an increase in blood level if that enzyme were inhibited)

CYP 1A	CYP 2C	CYP 2D6	CYP 3A3/4/5
clozapine	diazepam	amitriptyline	erythromycin
imipramine	amitriptyline	clomipramine	alprazolam
naproxen	clomipramine	desipramine	diazepam
theophylline		impipramine	HIV protease inhibitors
		paroxetine	cisapride
		haloperidol	chlorpheniramine
		risperidone	verapamil
		thioridazine	lovastatin
		codeine	methadone
		tamoxifen	sildenafil
		venlafaxine	tamoxifen
			trazodone

This is an adapted, partial list of CYP450 effects. The complete list is from David A. Flock-hart, M.D., Ph.D., Division of Clinical Pharmacology, Indiana University School of Medicine, and is available at http://medicine.iupui.edu/flockhart/.

TABLE 2. *Prices of Common Psychotropic Medications*

Prices shown are based on average wholesale for brand name medications, and the list wholesale pharmacy acquisition cost for generic medications. Prices vary from one pharmacy to another. These give an approximate sense of the cost of these medications, but cannot be used to determine what a specific medication will cost at your local pharmacy.

	Quantity (Tablet Size × Average)	Brand Name (Typical dose for 30 days)	Generic (Typical dose for 30 days)
ANTIPSYCHOTIC MEDICATIONS			
clozapine (Clozaril)*	100 mg × 4/day	$475.33	$388.35
fluphenazine (Prolixin)	10 mg/day	$ 80.31	$ 10.46
haloperidol (Haldol)	10 mg/day	N/A	$ 1.43
loxapine (Loxitane)	25 mg × 4/day	$266.40	$ 89.10
molindone (Moban)	25 mg × 4/day	$308.77	N/A
olanzapine (Zyprexa)	15 mg/day	$419.04	N/A
quetiapine (Seroquel)	300 mg × 2/day	$416.88	N/A
risperidone (Risperdal)	2 mg × 2/day	$240.60	N/A
thiothixene (Navane)	20 mg/day	$ 57.56	$ 20.20
trifluoperazine (Stelazine)	20 mg/day	$118.59	$ 24.95
ziprasidone (Geodon)	80 mg 2/day	$243.78	N/A
*plus week prescribing fee & weekly or biweekly white blood count			
(Long-acting injections)			
fluphenazine decanoate	12.5 mg × 2/month	$ 24.04	$ 14.83
haloperidol decanoate	100 mg/month	$ 66.18	$ 52.80
ANTIDEPRESSANT MEDICATIONS			
amitriptyline (Elavil, Endep)	150 mg/day	N/A	$ 2.17
bupropion (Wellbutrin)	150 mg × 2/day	$100.80	$ 46.33
bupropion SR (Wellbutrin SR)	150 mg × 2/day	$109.99	N/A
citalopram (Celexa)	40 mg × 1/day	$ 67.50	N/A
clomipramine (Anafranil)	75 mg × 2/day	$125.40	$ 17.82
desipramine (Norpramin, Pertofrane)	75 mg × 2/day	$ 36.00	$ 5.56
doxepin (Adapin, Sinequan)	100 mg × 2/day	$ 79.20	$ 7.66
fluoxetine (Prozac)	20 mg/day	$ 93.38	$ 10.00
imipramine (Tofranil)	150 mg/day	$ 89.54	$ 13.37
mirtazapine (Remeron)	45 mg × 1/day	$ 87.30	N/A
nefazodone (Serzone)	200 mg × 2/day	$ 94.79	N/A

(*continued*)

TABLE 2. *Continued*

	Quantity (Tablet Size × Average)	Brand Name (Typical dose for 30 days)	Generic (Typical dose for 30 days)
nortriptyline (Aventyl, Pamelor)	50 mg/day × 2day	$157.80	$ 4.75
paroxetine (Paxil)	20 mg/day	$ 81.48	N/A
sertraline (Zoloft)	100 mg/day × 2/day	$151.25	N/A
trazodone (Desyrel)	100 mg × 1/day	$105.90	$ 2.51
venlafaxine (Effexor)	75 mg × 2/day	$ 98.06	N/A
venlafaxine (Effexor XR)	75 mg × 2/day	$156.98	N/A
MOOD-STABILIZING MEDICATIONS			
carbamazepine (Tegretal)	200 mg × 4/day	$ 65.80	$ 15.30
oxcarbazepine (Trileptal)	600 mg × 2/day	$358.98	N/A
gabapentin (Neurontin)	400 mg 3/day	$134.73	N/A
lithium carbonate (Eskalith)	300 mg × 4/day	$ 24.42	$ 12.50
lithium controlled release (Eskalith CR)	450 mg × 3/day	$ 40.68	N/A
valproic acid (Depakene)	250 mg × 6/day	$320.40	$ 21.20
divalproex sodium (Depakote)	500 mg × 3/day	$157.61	N/A
ANTIANXIETY MEDICATIONS			
diazepam (Valium)	10 mg × 2/day	$ 90.60	$ 2.46
chlordiazepoxide (Librium)	25 mg × 4/day	$171.60	$ 7.13
oxazepam (Serax)	30 mg × 2/day	$141.17	$ 46.26
alprazolam (Xanex)	1 mg × 2/day	$ 92.40	$ 2.92
lorazepam (Ativan)	1 mg × 2/day	$ 64.80	$ 10.69
clonazepam (Klonopin)	1 mg × 2/day	$ 58.02	$ 6.77
buspirone (Buspar)	10 mg × 4/day	$184.56	$169.92
HYPNOTIC SLEEPING MEDICATIONS			
zaleplon (Sonata)	5 mg day.	$ 54.48	N/A
zolpidem (Ambien)	5 mg day	$ 54.60	N/A

A BRIEF DISCUSSION ABOUT MONEY

Those of us who prescribe, administer, and monitor psychotropic medications rarely consider how much they cost. Our clients, especially those who pay for their own medications, are painfully aware of the costs. The money spent on the medication is well worth it when measured against the increased suffering and dysfunction that would result if the medication were not available. Still, I think that we need to become more aware of the financial burden a prescription can impose on both the individual patient and the health care system. In 2000, 6% of the prescriptions written for Wisconsin Medical Assistance recipients were for antipsychotic medications, but these prescriptions cost 15% of the total pharmacy budget for the year. Sometimes, less expensive alternatives are just as effective as newer, brand-name medications. Both clozapine (Clozaril) and fluoxetine (Prozac) are now available as less expensive generic medications. There is still debate about whether generic medications are as good as brand-name medications. When I am prescribed medication by my physician, I generally use generic medications when they are available and I am comfortable prescribing generic medications for my patients. While some people report problems when switched from the brand name to the generic version of the same medication, this is very rare. Table 2 gives prices for both brand-name and generic psychotropic medications. As you can see, it is very common for clients to be prescribed medication that costs more than $100 per month.

3

Antipsychotic Medications

Antipsychotic medications are sometimes referred to as "major tranquilizers." This is a misleading term. While these medications all have calming effects, their major effect is to decrease hallucinations, delusions, and psychotic thinking. In general, other medications are safer and more effective if sedation is the sole aim. The term "neuroleptic" is also used for this class of medication, but this actually refers to a decrease in spontaneous and complex behaviors, which is a side effect rather than a positive effect of these medications. Over the past decade, new antipsychotic medications, often called atypical antipsychotics, has largely replaced the older or traditional antipsychotic medications. It is easier to understand how these new atypical medications work if you first understand something about how the traditional medications work. While this is not necessary in order to know how to use these medications, some understanding of how they work will make it easier to understand how they can help and what side effects they can cause.

HOW THEY WORK

Dopamine Pathways and Traditional Antipsychotic Medications

All of the traditional or older antipsychotic medications work by blocking dopamine receptors in the brain. Five different dopamine receptors have been discovered, labeled D_1 through D_5.

The traditional antipsychotic medications work by blocking the D_2 receptor. There are four major dopamine pathways in the brain, all of which are blocked by traditional antipsychotics. The first pathway starts in the brain stem and goes to the limbic system (mesolimbic pathway). Any chemical that decreases dopamine in the limbic system in the brain decreases psychotic symptoms. Any chemical that increases dopamine in this part of the brain, such as high-dose amphetamines, increases or causes psychotic symptoms. Antipsychotic medications are effective in decreasing psychotic symptoms because they block dopamine receptors in this limbic pathway.

Unfortunately, there are three other dopamine pathways. The second pathway starts in the brain stem and goes to the surface (cortex) of the frontal lobe of the brain (mesocortical pathway). Dopamine in the frontal cortex stimulates behavior, thought, expression, and motivation. When dopamine is blocked, there is decreased motivation, decreased spontaneity, and decreased ability to persist and follow through with things. Blocking dopamine in this area can cause side effects that exaggerate the "negative" symptoms of schizophrenia.

The third pathway starts in the brain stem and ends at the basal ganglion of the brain (nigrostriatal pathway), an area deep in the brain under the outer layer or cortex. This is the control system for the extrapyramidal motor system. Voluntary muscle movement starts in large pyramidal shaped cells in the surface (motor cortex) of the brain. The extrapyramidal motor system (outside the voluntary or pyramidal system) is involved in setting the correct muscle tension so that a person is not stiff, but also does not collapse. This is the system involved in making sure that movements are smooth. When dopamine in this area of the brain is blocked, you see extrapyramidal side effects (EPS), such as tremor, sudden muscle spasms (dystonias), and motor restlessness (akasthisia).

Finally, there is a dopamine pathway that tells the hypothalamus to stop making prolactin, one of the sex-related hormones. When dopamine in this pathway is blocked, the person's prolactin level goes up. This can cause breast enlargement and secretion of a milk-like liquid from breasts (in both men and women) along with other sexual side effects.

Joint Serotonin and Dopamine Blockers: Atypical Antipsychotic Medications

The atypical or newer antipsychotic medications block the D_2 receptors in the limbic pathways, while leaving the receptors in the other parts of the brain largely unaffected. These "atypical" antipsychotic medications accomplish this trick of selectively blocking dopamine receptors by using the brain's own self-regulation control system.

In some brain pathways, serotonin tells certain nerve cells to stop releasing dopamine. Serotonin acts like a brake on dopamine release. If these serotonin pathways are blocked, this brake is released and the nerve cells will release more dopamine. If *both* serotonin and dopamine are blocked at the same time, then more dopamine is released (because blocking serotonin increases dopamine release), but some of the dopamine receptors are also blocked and are therefore less sensitive to this extra dopamine. If the proportions of serotonin blockade and dopamine blockage are correct, then the final level of dopamine activity stays largely unchanged.

It turns out that there is no serotonin control system in the mesolimbic pathway, the one responsible for decreasing psychotic symptoms. There is a serotonin control system in the other three dopamine pathways. This means that if both dopamine and serotonin are blocked, there is dopamine blockade where we want it, but little or no dopamine blockade in the other pathways. By blocking both dopamine and serotonin at the same time, these medications act as though they selectively block dopamine in one part of the brain, while not affecting it in the rest of the brain. This of course depends on a very careful balance of the competing blockades, which makes this all more complicated than it sounds. As already mentioned, there are many different serotonin receptors. The one involved in the dopamine control system is $5HT_{2A}$. (The formal chemical name for serotonin is 5-hydroxytryptamine or 5HT. 5HT is shorthand for serotonin.) All of the atypical antipsychotic medications block both other serotonin receptors and nonserotonin receptors, which explains their differences from one another as well as some of their side effects.

ATYPICAL ANTIPSYCHOTIC MEDICATIONS

There are now five newer or "atypical" antipsychotic medications with more on the way. I strongly recommend one of these newer antipsychotic medications over the older, traditional medications for most people who need to start an antipsychotic or switch medications. I am more cautious about switching medications for someone doing well on a traditional antipsychotic, but over time I have recommended that even people doing well on an older medication should probably try one of the newer ones. There are a few people who seem to do better on the older medications than the newer ones; for people who do not respond to the new medications alone, a combination of both a traditional and an atypical antipsychotic may make sense. Someone who needs a long-acting injectable is currently limited to either haloperidol deconoate or fluphenazine deconoate, both older, traditional antipsychotics. It is expected that a long-acting risperidone will be available in the near future, and I expect that other long-acting atypicals will be available over the next few years. With these few exceptions, the atypical antipsychotic medications are now the preferred treatment for people who have psychotic symptoms.

Clozapine was the first of these new-generation antipsychotic medications to be marketed. Risperidone (Risperdal) was released in February 1994, olanzapine (Zyprexa) in 1996, quetiapine (Seroquel) in 1997, and ziprasidone (Geodon) in 2001. Several others are expected to be released in the next few years. All of these atypical antipsychotic medications block both dopamine D_2 and serotonin $5HT_{2A}$ receptors. Each of the new atypical antipsychotic medications has its own patterns of dopamine and serotonin blockade, and different patients respond to different medications. Unfortunately, there is no way to predict who will respond best to which medication. *This means that if someone does not respond well to one medication, it is well worth trying a second and then a third or a fourth before giving up and deciding that no medications work.*

The atypical antipsychotic medications have significant advantages over the older, traditional medications. All of these atypical antipsychotic medications have fewer extrapyramidal (muscle-related) side effects than traditional medications. These newer medications also seem less likely to cause tardive dyskinesia. Fewer people taking these atypical antipsychotics develop what is called a "dysphoric response," or feeling "zombie-like," a side effect sometimes felt a few days after starting a traditional antipsychotic medication. People with a dysphoric reaction may report that they feel terrible but may not be able to describe what the feeling specifically is. Finally, the atypical antipsychotics are effective in some people who did not respond to older medications. They not only work in more people, they work better in many people, even those who had some improvement on the older medications. While this increased effectiveness is best documented for clozapine, it seems to be true for the other atypicals as well.

All of these atypical medications are much more expensive than the older medications. This enormous increase in the cost of medication has had a major financial impact on mental health budgets. When atypical medications were first introduced, there was active debate about whether the advantages of the medications justified their costs. While cost continues to be a major concern, it is now clear that the new atypical antipsychotic medications are both more effective than the older drugs and have side effects that most people find easier to live with. Atypical antipsychotic medications are now the accepted standard for the initial treatment of people with a psychotic illness.

TRADITIONAL ANTIPSYCHOTIC MEDICATIONS

All of the older or traditional antipsychotic medications work by blocking receptor sites in the brain that are usually stimulated by dopamine. All of the traditional antipsychotic medications are equally effective, but they vary in potency—that is, they all do an equally good job, but it takes different amounts of each medication for them to be equally effective. A 100-mg dose of Thorazine is equal in effectiveness to a 2-mg dose of Haldol.

The different traditional antipsychotic medications do have somewhat different side effects, although this is a matter of degree rather than kind. In general, the high-potency antipsychotic medications (such as Prolixin, Haldol, and Navane) are both safer and better tolerated by most people than low-potency medications like Thorazine. The high-potency medications are relatively less sedating; cause fewer anticholinergic side effects (anticholinergic refers to a medication that blocks the cholinergic part of the nervous system) such as dry mouth, constipation, and blurred vision; and cause less postural hypotension (a drop in blood pressure from sitting down or standing up too quickly). They are also somewhat safer than low-potency medications. However, they more commonly cause extrapyramidal side effects (EPS), such as tremor and motor restlessness. Medications such as benztropine (Cogentin) can decrease EPS effects. Unfortunately, such medications do not always take away all of the EPS side effects, and they can have side effects of their own.

INDICATIONS FOR USE

As noted before, a comprehensive assessment and diagnosis should be made before starting any medication. Medications should not be given just because a person is upset or because he or she is psychotic. Delirium needs to be ruled out first. In addition, medical illness or drug intoxication need to be considered, as these may present as psychosis.

1. *Psychotic Agitation*

The antipsychotic medications are just that—antipsychotic. They decrease psychotic symptoms no matter what the cause. Psychosis from schizophrenia, mania, dementia and other neurological disorders, or psychosis from hallucinogenic drugs will all generally respond. Unfortunately, the antipsychotic effects can take days to weeks.

These medications also have immediate sedative and calming effects separate from their antipsychotic effects. The decrease in psychosis often seen within a few minutes after taking an antipsychotic medication is an effect of sedation rather than a specific antipsychotic effect. In the first few hours, an antipsychotic like haloperidol and a sedative antianxiety medication like lorazepam (Ativan) will have very similar effects. Calming someone down by listening and supporting them can also have a similar effect. Anything that helps calm a very agitated person down will help them become more organized and less psychotic. There is also a direct antipsychotic effect that is very different than just sedation, but this takes several days or weeks to become apparent.

In the past, people with a diagnosis of schizophrenia who became psychotic and agitated were often given repeated doses of 2–5 mg of Haldol by either liquid concentrate, pills, or injection until they calmed down. Research shows that waiting after one of two doses of these medications will decrease agitation and psychotic symptoms as fast as higher dose strategies. When additional sedation is required, a combination of an antipsychotic medication and an antianxiety medication such as lorazepam (Ativan) is safe, effective, and more comfortable for the patient than administering a high dose of the antipsychotic medication.

The atypical medications are rapidly replacing older medications as the treatment of choice in calming people who are both agitated and psychotic. There are important differences between the newer medications; each has its own advantages and disadvantages. In general, it appears that as a group they cause the same calming effect as older medications but with less behavioral inhibition. This behavioral inhibition was really a side effect from the older medications and is often uncomfortable for the patient. While helping someone calm down might be useful in an emergency when someone is out of control, being made to feel "wooden" and losing spontaneity becomes a problem when the same medication has to be taken for a long period of time. This and other side effects are often so uncomfortable that people given traditional antipsychotics in an emergency may be less willing to take them later. The atypical antipsychotics appear useful in an emergency, but since they are much less of a "chemical straight jacket" they must be used somewhat differently.

Ziprasidone, olanzapine, and risperidone are all effective in calming agitated psychotic people rapidly, and all seem well tolerated. All are expected to soon be available in a short-acting injectable form for emergency use. Olanzapine can safely be given at a full dose (5–20 mg). Risperidone (Risperdal) and ziprasidone (Geodon) are usually started in somewhat less than a full dose to decrease side effects. While this makes starting the medication a bit more complicated, it does not seem to decrease their effectiveness in emergency situations. Quetiapine (Seroquel) is the most sedating of the atypical antipsychotics (with the exception of clozapine, which is never started as an emergency medication). Quetiapine is usually started at a low dose (25 mg twice a day) and then increased every day or two, but in an emergency it can be started a bit higher and given more frequently. The biggest problem with starting quetiapine at too high a dose is dizziness and the risk of falls. At times, the sedation of quetiapine can be useful, but in general it is probably less useful as an emergency medication for people who are psychotic.

In general, if additional sedation is needed, adding a benzo-diazepine such as lorazepam (Ativan) can calm someone safely and rapidly.

2. *Schizophrenia*

Symptoms of schizophrenia can be divided into positive symptoms (hallucinations and delusions), negative symptoms (apathy, social withdrawal, loss of spontaneity, lack of pleasure in things), and cognitive symptoms (problems with memory, making decisions). While positive symptoms are more dramatic and more clearly associated with "being crazy," negative and cognitive symptoms cause more disability and are more associated with poor quality of life. It is possible to hold a job while you believe you are God or hear voices, but it is very difficult to hold a job if you cannot motivate yourself to work or if you cannot remember what you are supposed to do. Traditional antipsychotic medications are generally very effective for positive and disorganized symptoms but less effective for negative or cognitive symptoms. The atypical antipsychotic medications seem to work on positive, negative, and cognitive symptoms.

Initial treatment for schizophrenia is targeted on symptom control and helping the person reestablish control over his or her behavior. This might mean helping the person become stable enough to leave the hospital or recover from a crisis. Older, traditional antipsychotic medications were once used in the hospital in somewhat higher than normal doses to help the person get through the crisis period as rapidly as possible. With the traditional antipsychotic medications, it was thought that more was better, despite the lack of research to support this idea. The balance between the need for speed and the risk of uncomfortable side effects must always be considered, but for someone in a hospital, erring a bit high is sometimes thought to be better than erring too low.

It is extremely important to decrease side effects as much as possible if we do not want people to discontinue their medication. You can often decrease the side effects caused by traditional antipsychotic medications by just lowering the dose. Research suggests that many people—even those with severe long-term illnesses—do well with much lower doses of traditional antipsychotic medications than previously thought, especially if they are monitored closely and given additional medication during periods of relapse. Haloperidol at 5 mg/day seems as effective as higher doses for many people with schizophrenia—at least those with fairly recent onset of the illness—and causes many fewer side effects.

The situation is more complicated with the atypical antipsychotics. With risperidone, less is better, and people often do better with fewer side effects on 4 mg/day of risperidone than on higher doses. With quetiapine, on the other hand, more is often better. It seems a more effective antipsychotic medication as the dose is raised above 400 or 600 mg/day, and it is now being used above 1,000 mg/day with few problems. With quetiapine, it appears that the side effects do not get worse with higher doses. The dose strategy must be individualized for each medication and for each client. With olanzapine, more might be more effective, but higher doses also lead to more side effects.

The majority of people with schizophrenia will have a relapse if they discontinue their antipsychotic medication. Some people with schizophrenia whose illness has stabilized over a number of years and who are now approaching middle age may remain stable even without medication. It is unclear how many people can safely discontinue their medication after years of treatment, or how to predict who will do well and who will not. What is clear is that at least in the first five to ten years of the illness, few people with schizophrenia will do well without regular use of antipsychotic medication.

Attempts have also been made to use a targeted medication strategy where the person does not stay on medication but restarts medication rapidly at the first early sign of a relapse. For most people with schizophrenia, targeted medication strategies lead to more relapses, more re-hospitalizations, and poorer functioning.

Most people with schizophrenia do not relapse immediately if they discontinue antipsychotic medication. Research has suggested that a person with schizophrenia who discontinues medication has around a 10% chance of relapsing during the first month. Of those people who do not relapse during the first month off medication, approximately 10% will relapse in the second month, and so on, with around 10% of the remaining people relapsing every month they are off medication. Some people will go many months before relapsing, but this brief period of stability does not mean that medication is no longer needed.

3. *Manic Depression—Acute Mania Phase*
All of the antipsychotic medications seem to be useful in treating mania. Research demonstrates olanzapine's effectiveness with mania. It also can be started at a full dose right at the beginning, and the dose can rapidly be raised to even higher doses if necessary. Risperidone (Risperdal) and ziprasidone (Geodon) both are useful in treating mania, especially as a way of increasing the effectiveness of a mood-stabilizing medication like lithium or Depakote, and of increasing behavioral control during the first few days or weeks. Quetiapine (Seroquel) has significant mood-stabilizing antimanic effects and its sedative side effects can be useful in calming someone who is agitated or manic. Unfortunately, quetiapine must be started at a low dose and increased over several days or weeks. This makes it less useful in an emergency, unless the person is already on one of these medications and the dose can just be increased. Clozapine in particular is an extremely effective mood-stabilizing medication; despite all of its many side effects, it has a role for people with manic depression who have not responded to anything else. It has many side effects, requires regular blood tests, and must be started slowly and increased over time. Despite its effective-

ness as an ongoing medication, clozapine has no role in an emergency situation.

Risperidone, olanzapine, and ziprasidone are all useful in the emergency control of people who are manic. While atypical antipsychotics are now increasingly used as the treatment of choice, there may still be a role for the older medications as well. The traditional approach has been to use traditional antipsychotics in a moderate to large dose (e.g., haloperidol at 5 mg once or twice a day) to establish rapid behavioral control until lithium or Depakote has had time to become effective. When more sedation and behavioral control are needed, an antipsychotic medication can be combined with a benzodiazepine (clonazepam or lorazepam) rather than increasing the dose of the antipsychotic. This often allows for behavioral control with fewer side effects. It was once believed that antipsychotic medications were the most effective way to rapidly control the behavior of people with mania. Now, benzodiazepines are being used more frequently to establish behavioral control in people who are hypomanic but not psychotic.

4. *Organic Brain Syndrome (OBS)*
Antipsychotic medication is often beneficial in very low doses (olanzapine 2.5 mg hs [before bed] or risperidone 0.5 to 1.5 mg). Doses should be kept low, as higher doses can cause confusion and behavioral problems to worsen, especially in elderly people and people with dementia. Antipsychotic medication can help control both problematic behavior and emotional lability in some people with OBS. Medications should be used only after the medical work-up of the OBS is completed and the diagnosis is firmly established. Again, there are important differences between the various atypical medications, but all are effective in this client population and all have been used.

5. *Delusional (Psychotic) Depression*
People who are psychotic or suffer delusional depression initially respond much better to the combination of antipsychotic and antidepressant medications than to antidepressants

alone. Once the client has begun to respond, the antipsychotic medication can be tapered and then discontinued,
leaving the antidepressant for maintenance therapy. Except
in very rare cases, antipsychotic medications should not be
used as maintenance medication for people who have previously had a psychotic depression but who are not currently
psychotic. Also, some very agitated depressed people will
have a faster feeling of relief and faster agitation reduction if
low-dose antipsychotic medications are initially used along
with the antidepressants. Again, these medications should be
used only for short periods of time in these depressed people.

Nonagitated, nondelusional depressed people are often
made worse by traditional antipsychotic medications. Too
high a dose of traditional antipsychotic medication can trigger depression in any client. The atypical antipsychotic medications seem much less likely than the traditional antipsychotics
to cause depression, and some of the newer medications may
even have direct antidepressant activity.

6. *Drug-induced Psychosis*
Some drug-induced psychosis can be handled by allowing
the person to let it "wear off" in a low stimulus environment.
LSD can often be handled with emotional support without
antipsychotic medication. Other drug-induced psychosis does
require pharmacological intervention and can typically respond to antipsychotic medications. There are some potentially dangerous drug-drug interactions. For example, very
high doses of PCP (phencyclidine) can cause rapid unstable
changes in blood pressure that are made much worse with
antipsychotic medications. Deaths occurred when orally in-
gested high-dose PCP intoxication was rapidly treated with
high-dose chlorpromazine. This is only a risk during the very
initial acute phase of intoxication when the drug levels are
at their highest. Despite this unusual risk, antipsychotics for
the most part are safe and effective when used for drug-
induced psychosis. Acutely, benzodiazepines are useful in

decreasing agitation, but for more persistent psychosis the antipsychotic medications are indicated.

A Word about Cigarette Smoking and Antipsychotics

Cigarette smoking induces (increases the activity of) the enzymes that break down antipsychotic (and many other) medications. This means that smokers may need a higher dose of medication than nonsmokers. It also means that if someone *stops* smoking, his or her serum level of medication will increase and medication side effects may develop. This affects some medications more than others, depending on how the particular medication is broken down in the liver. For example, smoking can have a significant effect on clozapine levels, but usually has only a very small effect on risperidone levels.

Other Drug-Drug Interactions with Antipsychotic Medications

There are potentially dangerous interactions for some of the antipsychotics with many of the medications used in the treatment of HIV. For example, Norvir and Kaletra both inhibit the enzyme that are used to metabolize clozapine, olanzapine, and risperdidone. When used together, these medications should be used at ¼ to ½ of the normal dose. Some of the other medications used to treat HIV also have important drug-drug interactions with antipsychotics.

SPECIFICS OF USE FOR ATYPICAL ANTIPSYCHOTIC MEDICATIONS

Clozapine (Clozaril)

Clozapine is the most effective antipsychotic now available. Because it has so many side effects, other medications should be tried first, but anyone with schizophrenia who continues to have major problems after trying two or three of the other newer antipsychotics should try clozapine before deciding that medications do not work at all. Clozapine is also an extremely effective mood stabilizer and can be used to treat people with bipolar disorders who have not responded to mood stabilizers. Finally, like the other atypical antipsychotic medications, clozapine seems much more effective with the cognitive and negative symptoms of schizophrenia than traditional medications.

Side Effects. Clozapine has many side effects, some dangerous and others not dangerous but difficult to live with. Sedation and weight gain are the two biggest, most common side effects with clozapine. The sedation often improves over time but can continue to be a major problem. Not everyone on clozapine gains weight, but the average weight gain after a year is more than 20 pounds, which means that some people gain much less than this, but some people gain much more. Drooling, especially at night, is a problem for some people. Clozapine has strong anticholinergic side effects (dry mouth, blurred vision, constipation) and can cause orthostatic blood pressure drops (a sudden blood pressure drop when the person stands up suddenly). Other side effects include fever, headache, nausea, and rapid pulse. While these side effects can be uncomfortable, they are not usually dangerous.

Clozapine is associated with fatal heatstroke. *In very hot weather people taking clozapine should try to find a place to stay that is cool or air-conditioned. They should also take care to drink fluids and avoid excessive exercise.* Some of these fatalities from heatstroke have occurred in medically healthy young men who would not typically be thought of as being at high risk, but dehydration and exercise increase the risk.

In higher doses, clozapine causes seizures more frequently than the other antipsychotic medications. While seizures can be extremely frightening, they are not life-threatening. An anticonvulsant such as Depakote is often used along with higher doses of clozapine to decrease the risk of seizures.

The most common medically serious side effect from clozapine is diabetes. People tend to develop adult onset diabetes as they get older. This is more frequent for people who are overweight and, as already mentioned, clozapine can cause significant weight gain. While there is some debate about this, it also seems that people taking clozapine (and olanzapine) are more likely to develop diabetes even if they do not gain weight. Diabetes is associated with a large number of serious problems, including heart disease, stroke, blindness and kidney disease.

Most seriously, 1% of people taking clozapine will develop agranulocytosis (they will stop making white blood cells). If this is discovered in time and the medication is stopped, the client can recover without difficulty. If this drop in white blood cells is not discovered, the person can die from infections that he or she can no longer fight. There were at least 13 reported deaths from clozapine between 1990 and 1996, even with regular blood testing. Most cases of agranulocytosis occur 6–18 weeks after starting clozapine. Currently, anyone starting clozapine is required to get a weekly count of white blood cells to ensure that they are still being produced. More frequent monitoring is required for people whose total white cell count decreases to 3,000–3,500 cells. Anyone with a total white count below 3,000 or a granulocyte count (mature white cell count) of less than 1,500 must immediately discontinue clozapine. In the United States, for the first six months a person can get only a week of medication at a time and cannot receive the next week's medication without first obtaining a blood test. After six months, people are allowed to decrease their blood tests to every other week. Unfortunately, this means that people who do not want to put up with the hassle of weekly or biweekly tests cannot benefit from the medication. It also means that clozapine can be prescribed only when an organized monitoring system is in place.

Specifics of Use. To decrease the risk of seizures and other side effects, clozapine is usually started at 12.5 or 25 mg/day and then increased by 25 mg every three days until a dose of

300–450 mg is reached by the end of two to three weeks. Subsequent increases should be at no more than 25 mg at a time, with increases no more frequent than every two days. The majority of people respond to 300–600 mg/day. The maximum dose is 900 mg/day, but seizures are more frequent above 600 mg. It is now suggested that anyone taking clozapine in high doses also take divalproex sodium (Depakote) to decrease the risk of seizures. Depakote is commonly used in psychiatry as a mood stabilizer (discussed later), but its primary use in medicine is as an anticonvulsant. It is recommended that clozapine be taken twice a day, but in the lower end of the dose range it seems safe and effective to give it once a day if side effects are carefully monitored. Some data suggests that clozapine is more effective if the serum level is above 350 ng/ml.

Clozapine may take a long time to be effective. Some people who do not respond after four weeks at a full dose will show a later response, and many people who initially have only a partial response will respond better after taking the medication for six months or more. If someone does not respond to clozapine, they may respond to a combination of clozapine and a low dose of another antipsychotic. There is also the suggestion that some of the side effects of clozapine, especially weight gain and drooling, can be reduced if quetiapine or another atypical antipsychotic is added, and the dose of clozapine is decreased.

Drug-Drug Interactions. Caffeine is reported to increase clozapine levels in some patients, while smoking can lower them. SSRI-type antidepressants can increase clozapine levels, and anticonvulsants, including valproate, can decrease them. Medications used outside of psychiatry can also affect clozapine levels. For example, the antibiotic erythromycin and the anti-ulcer medication cimetidine can increase clozapine levels to potentially dangerous levels. There may be a risk in combining clozapine with a benzodiazepine, especially if the dose is rapidly increased. There have been at least seven reported incidents of people stopping breathing after they were given a benzodiazepine while on clozapine. Given the number of people who have had no problems taking clozapine and a benzodiazepine, the risk of stopping breathing appears very low. Confusion, sedation, and increased salivation from the combination have also been reported.

Cost. Clozapine is very expensive, although the price has dropped now that its patent has run out and generic versions have been introduced. A typical dose of brand-name Clozaril at 400 mg/day costs approximately $440 per month. The same dose of the generic equivalent costs approximately $232 per month (based on charges to Wisconsin Medicaid). To this must be added the cost of the weekly or biweekly blood tests. I feel that there is little reason not to use a less expensive generic version when available. Some concerns have been raised that the generic and brand-name products may have slightly different pharmacokinetic properties. This means that as one switches from clozapine manufactured by one company to that produced by another, there *may* be slight differences in serum levels—in some patients this may be clinically important. This problem is currently hotly debated and I have not seen any difficulty for people who are switched from a brand-name to a generic medication. Some physicians and some patients have continued on the more expensive brand-name version because they are uncomfortable risking any change when a person with a serious illness is improving. The pharmaceutical company involved, in an effort to maintain market share, has tried to reinforce the idea that staying on the brand-name medication decreases risk. I think what makes more sense is to pay careful attention to any changes in symptoms or ability to function as one switches between clozapine made by different companies and to adjust the dose up or down as needed. Clozapine blood levels may help, especially if you knew the blood level both before and after the switch. While some doctors suggest getting these before and after blood levels as part of the routine of switching, I do not feel this is necessary and would rather just follow clinical status.

Risperidone (Risperdal)

Risperidone was the second new-generation atypical antipsychotic medication to be marketed. When used in the recommended dose range of 4–6 mg/day, it has relatively few extrapyramidal side effects, which gives it a major advantage over older medications. While not as effective as clozapine, it seems to work for some people who have not responded to traditional antipsychotics. It also seems more effective than traditional antipsychotics in decreasing negative and cognitive symptoms. Finally, risperidone may also have some antidepressant activity.

Side Effects. The main advantage of risperidone is that it has relatively few side effects. Weight gain is a problem, although less of a risk with risperidone than with clozapine or olanzapine. Risperidone commonly causes elevation of prolactin, a hormone that can cause various sexual side effects, including amenorrhea in women and breast enlargement in both men and women. Orthostatic hypotension (sudden drops in blood pressure when the client stands quickly) may be a problem especially in older people who can fall as a result. Insomnia and agitation are more often reported rather than the sedation seen with most other antipsychotic medications. Akathisia (motor restlessness) is somewhat more common than with the other atypical antipsychotics, but it is much less frequent and less severe than with the traditional antipsychotic medications. Other potential side effects include nausea and a runny nose. Any medication can cause agranulocytosis (sudden block in the production of white blood cells), but the incidence of this with risperidone appears to be very low and no special blood tests or monitoring are required. The incidence of seizures also seems very low.

Specifics of Use. A full dose of risperidone for most people with schizophrenia is 4–6 mg/day. Two mg/day seems less effective, at least for most people with schizophrenia, and the frequency of extrapyramidal side effects, especially akathisia, increase as the dose is raised above 4 mg/day. Raising the dose above 6 mg/day increases the risk of akathisia and other extrapyramidal side effects considerably with little apparent increase in effectiveness for most people. Risperidone has a half-life of around 20 hours, which means that most people can take it once a day without problems.

In elderly demented people, very small amounts of risperidone (0.5–1.5 mg/day) are often useful in controlling psychotic symptoms and agitation. It has begun to replace haloperidol as the preferred antipsychotic for these people. Orthostatic hypotension and falls are a potential problem, but the lack of anticholinergic side effects, relatively little sedation, and few EPS effects are all major advantages.

Cost. While risperidone is an expensive medication, it is the least expensive of the atypical antipsychotics. A standard dose of 4 mg/day has an average wholesale cost of $2,927 per year.

Olanzapine (Zyprexa)

Olanzapine was the third atypical antipsychotic to be marketed in the United States. It was designed to be more "clozapine-like" than risperidone and shares some of clozapine's advantages and disadvantages. It seems effective and very well tolerated. It works for people who have not responded to other medications and seems effective on negative and cognitive symptoms as well as positive symptoms.

Side Effects. It has a low incidence of motor side effects when used below 10 mg/day. Akathisia (motor restlessness) becomes more of a problem when the dose is raised above this, especially when raised above 20 mg/day. Like risperidone, it has an extremely low incidence of blood dyscrasias or seizures.

A big problem with olanzapine is weight gain. Average weight gain varies from study to study but seems to be around 20 pounds over six months. This means some people gain very little, while others may gain more than 20 pounds. Olanzapine causes significantly more weight gain than ziprasidone or risperidone but less than clozapine. The weight gain seems to be caused by carbohydrate craving. Not everyone gains weight and diet control and exercise can help prevent a weight problem from starting. Much of the weight gain, when it occurs, happens in the first few weeks after olanzapine is started. Informing people about the risk of weight gain, early monitoring of weight, and direct suggestions about weight control strategies can help. It is important to educate the person and support weight control efforts but not to blame the patient for weight gain. The weight gain associated with olanzapine and the other atypical medications is often very difficult to fight. The initial period of weight gain often occurs while the person is struggling to overcome the effects of their mental illness, and it is frequently accompanied by poverty and restricted activity, which compound the problem. Diabetes is also a concern. There is an increased risk of diabetes with weight gain, but there also seems to be an increased incidence of adult onset diabetes in people taking olanzapine (and clozapine), even without weight gain.

Other possible side effects include drowsiness, dizziness, dry mouth, and orthostatic hypotension. Agitation, nausea, and indigestion are rarer but have also been reported. Olanzapine does not cause the elevation of prolactin seen in risperidone or traditional antipsychotic medications and seems to have fewer sexual side effects than older medications. Increases in liver enzymes have been reported but are rarely a significant problem.

Specifics of Use. A typical dose of olanzapine for someone with schizophrenia is 10–20 mg/day. In a healthy adult, 10 mg can be given as the starting dose, although there will be less initial sedation if 5 mg is used first and then increased after a day or two. EPSE (motor) side effects, especially akathisia, become more common in doses above 20 mg/day. It is safe to increase the dose of olanzapine to 30 or 40 mg or even higher, but relatively few people will respond to these very high doses if they have not responded to 20 mg. Olanzapine has significant mood-stabilizing properties and can be used as initial treatment for someone who is manic.

Cost. Olanzapine is both one of the most expensive and one of the most commonly used antipsychotic medications. As a result, it has become a very significant cost issue for medicaid and other authorities responsible for funding mental health care. The average wholesale cost for a 15 mg/day of olanzapine is $5,098 per year.

Quetiapine (Seroquel)

Quetiapine was released in October 1997. It seems both effective and well tolerated. It has essentially no extrapyramidal side effects and fairly low anticholinergic side effects. It also causes no prolactin elevation, which suggests that it might have fewer sexual side effects than some of the other antipsychotic medications. It is more sedating than olanzapine, but much less sedating than clozapine.

Side Effects. It causes a slight increase in pulse and a temporary release of enzymes from the liver into the blood. This increase in circulating liver enzymes is reported as an abnormality in some tests of liver function. These effects are seldom problematic. Orthostatic hypotension (drop in blood pressure when standing suddenly) is a problem for some people. Weight gain may also be a problem for some people taking quetiapine, as it is for all the atypical antipsychotics.

The weight gain with quetiapine is less than that caused by olanzapine and probably about the same as that caused by risperidone.

Animal testing has suggested that quetiapine might be associated with an increased frequency of developing cataracts. It is unclear if this is really a problem in normal clinical use, but the manufacturer's recommendation is that people taking quetiapine get baseline and then regular eye exams. I feel that this is more a medical or legal issue than a clinical issue. There is no clinical data from its use with people that the risk of cataracts is significantly more than with many other medications. I do feel that everyone should get a regular eye exam, whether or not they are taking medication.

Specifics of Use. Quetiapine has a short half-life of six hours, which suggests it should be taken twice a day when possible. It is usually started at 25 mg twice a day, increasing rapidly every day or two. There is more dizziness and sedation when a higher initial dose is used, but the dizziness disappears over a few days. Quetiapine has a reputation for being less effective than the other atypical antipsychotic medications, but this is related to using too low a dose. With quetiapine, more is better. A minimal effective dose for treatment of schizophrenia is 400 mg/day, and it is often more effective in doses of 600 mg/day and above. It seems that the sedation and other side effects do not increase as the dose is raised above 400 mg/day, but the medication seems much more effective in higher doses. The formal FDA maximum dose is 750 mg/day, but some clinicians are using it in doses above 1,000 mg/day with few problems and increased effectiveness.

Quetiapine also seems a well-tolerated effective medication for people with borderline personality disorders who often experience mood lability and who have symptoms of thought disorder under stress. It is safe, nonaddicting, and can provide some sedation and help calm people who are having problems organizing their thinking.

Cost. Quetiapine is one of the more expensive antipsychotic medications now in use. At 600 mg/day, the average wholesale price for quetiapine is $5,072 per year. When doses of quetiapine above 600 mg/day are used, the price becomes even higher.

Ziprasidone (Geodon)

Ziprasidone became available in early 2001. It is the first atypical antipsychotic that is "weight neutral." While some people may gain or lose a few pounds, most people will have no weight change from the medication. It is also activating for most people, rather than sedating like all of the other antipsychotics. Ziprasidone also causes no prolactin elevation, which means that it should have fewer sexual side effects. While there is less research data on ziprasidone because it is new, it seems generally as effective as the other atypical antipsychotic medications that have been in use for a longer period of time. We will need to wait for more experience and more data, but it may have antidepressant as well as antipsychotic effects. Ziprasidone is a short-acting medication that is recommended to be taken twice a day, preferably with meals.

Side Effects. While it may cause sedation in some people when first started, the most common initial side effects of ziprasidone are agitation and insomnia. This can be a particular problem for people who are already agitated and having trouble sleeping. People are more comfortable and more likely to stay on ziprasidone if a benzodiazepine like lorazepam is used to treat these side effects, especially in the first few days after ziprasidone is started. Nausea is sometimes reported, especially after the medication is first started. So far, ziprasidone seems to have relatively few EPS effects, but like risperidone this is likely to be more of a problem as the dose is increased.

The biggest concern with ziprasidone is that it increases the time that it takes for the heart to prepare itself for its next contraction. After every heartbeat, the heart "repolarizes" or resets itself. If a new heartbeat starts during this repolarization period, it is possible that the heart will start quivering instead of having an organized contraction. If this starts and the heart cannot reset itself, the person can suddenly and without warning drop dead. The time from the beginning of the heartbeat to the end of the repolarization period is called the QT interval. Since it is naturally shorter when the heart beats faster and longer when the heart beats slower, this is corrected for the heart rate. This corrected measurement is called the QTc interval. It is a theoretical risk that heart quivering can start at any time, but it is more likely if the QTc interval is longer. With a longer QTc interval, it is more likely that the next contraction will start before the heart is ready for it. Any medication that increases the QTc interval increases this risk of sudden death. A large number of commonly used medications increase the QTc interval. Ziprasidone also increases the QTc interval, and therefore increases the risk of sudden death. This risk of sudden death is greater if the person has heart damage or is taking other medications that also increase the QTc interval.

The question is how big is this risk? The risk is certainly real, but it also seems very small. Initial research involving 4,500 people showed that the incidence of heart problems was about the same as other medications, which are considered pretty safe. There is a lot of very technical debate, in part fueled by competition between the pharmaceutical companies. My feeling is that if someone has other reasons for concern, such as being older, being very obese, having known heart disease, or being on other medications known to have a strong effect on prolonging QTc interval, then an EKG should be obtained before starting ziprasidone. Otherwise I see the risk as low and an EKG as unnecessary. While there is probably some theoretical but very small risk of sudden death with ziprasidone, the long-term risk of heart problems is less than the other antipsychotic medications because it does not cause weight gain or diabetes, both of which are associated with heart disease and other cardiovascular problems.

Specifics of Use. The FDA recommends that ziprasidone be started at 20 mg twice a day and increased as needed up to a maximum dose of 80 mg twice a day. The research data suggests that 20 mg twice a day is not likely to be effective, and there is little problem with starting at a higher dose. I typically start a healthy young adult at 40 mg twice a day. It appears that the antidepressant effect of ziprasidone is only seen at the higher end of the dose range, 80 mg twice a day. Because of concern about its effects on the heart, it is not recommended above a total of 160 mg/day. The medication is better absorbed with food, so, while it is safe to take it on an empty stomach, it is recommended to be taken with meals. Since it often causes agitation, it makes sense to take it at breakfast and dinner, rather than right before bed when other antipsychotic medications are commonly taken. It is a very short-acting medication. There is little experience with giving it once rather than twice a day. While twice a day is clearly recommended, once a day seems to be effective as well.

Since ziprasidone is activating rather than sedating, the early sedation that we have come to expect from other antipsychotics is usually not present. This sometimes leads to the feeling that the medication is not working. At other times, sleep problems or agitation can be a problem. Combining ziprasidone with a benzodiazepine like lorazepam, especially when starting treatment, can decrease this early agitation and insomnia.

Cost. While ziprasidone is expensive, it is among the least expensive of the atypical antipsychotic medications. The average wholesale price for ziprasidone at 80 mg twice a day is $2,966 per year.

Iloperidone (not yet available)

As we learn more about how antipsychotic medications work, it becomes possible for the chemists to design new molecules that work in very specific ways. Iloperidone is now being tested, and, if continued research supports early findings, it should be available within the next year or two. It has a similar mechanism of action to the other atypical antipsychotic medications in that it blocks both dopamine and serotonin receptors. Because of its effects on different serotonin receptors, it appears to cause little or no weight gain, little EPS effects, little sedation, and little effect on heart function. It promises to be an effective antipsychotic medication with fewer side effects than currently available medications.

Aripiprazole (not yet available)

Aripiprizole is a new medication that works through a different mechanism than currently available antipsychotic medications. It blocks serotonin receptors similar to other atypical antipsychotics. In addition, it both blocks but also partially stimulates dopamine receptors, instead of just blocking these receptors as current medications all do. The hope is that this will allow a response with more normal brain function.

In early research, it appears to be effective with few side effects. As with the other antipsychotics that should be made available within the next year or two, it appears to cause little or no weight gain, little EPS effects, little sedation, and little effect on heart function.

SPECIFICS OF USE FOR TRADITIONAL ANTIPSYCHOTIC MEDICATIONS

Chlorpromazine (Thorazine)

Chlorpromazine was the first effective antipsychotic medication. Initially introduced to the United States in 1953, it revolutionized the treatment of people with schizophrenia. While it

TABLE 3. *Advantages and Disadvantages of Atypical Antipsychotic Medications*

	Advantages	Disadvantages
Clozapine (Clozaril)	• Works when other medications do not • Works better than other medications • Very little EPS effects	• Weekly blood tests • Agranulocytosis • Sedation, drooling, weight gain, diabetes, seizures
Olanzapine (Zyprexa)	• Well tolerated • Can be started at full dose • Rapid control of symptoms • No prolactin elevation	• Weight gain • Diabetes
Quetiapine (Seroquel)	• Well tolerated • Very little EPS effects • No prolactin elevation	• Dose must be increased over time—400–600 mg/day needed to be effective • Sedation • Weight gain
Risperidone (Risperdal)	• Less sedation • Less weight gain • Less diabetes	• Prolactin elevation • EPS effects with higher doses • Dose must increase over few days
Ziprasidone (Geodon)	• No weight gain • Not sedating • No prolactin elevation	• Heart conduction abnormalities • Agitation/insomnia

TABLE 4. *Side Effects of Atypical Antipsychotic Medications*

	EPS Effects	Sedation	Weight Gain	Orthostatic Hypotension	Anticholinergic Effects
Clozapine	+/−	++++	++++	++++	++++
Olanzapine	+	+++	+++	+	++
Quetiapine	+/−	+++	++	+	+
Risperidone	++	++	+	++	+
Ziprasidone	++	+	−	++	+

Key: +Mild   ++Moderate   +++Major   ++++Severe   +/−Minimal   −none still has a role, it is very sedating and causes people to feel "drugged" or "zombie-like" and is now rarely used as a primary medication. At times, this sedation makes it a useful medication to use before bed to promote sleep.

Side Effects. The most sedating antipsychotics, such as chlorpromazine (Thorazine) and thioridazine (Mellaril) also have the most anticholinergic side effects, including dry mouth, blurred vision, constipation, and occasional urinary retention (an inability to urinate, especially in older men). These antipsychotics also have the highest frequency of orthostatic hypotension (an abrupt drop in blood pressure when the client stands up). At the same time, chlorpromazine and thioridazine are much less likely to cause EPS effects than the traditional high-potency antipsychotics like haloperidol (Haldol) or fluphenazine (Prolixin) and therefore there is less need to use antiparkinsonian medications to control them. Chlorpromazine occasionally causes extreme sensitivity to sunlight and can cause cataracts in the eye.

Specifics of Use. A typical dose range for people who are psychotic is 400–1,500 mg/day in divided doses. It is commonly said that 400 mg/day is a minimal antipsychotic dose for people with schizophrenia, although there is increasing interest in studying the effectiveness of very low doses. There is little research supporting the use of more than 600–700 mg/day. In the past, injections of chlorpromazine were commonly used to sedate very agitated people. There are safer and more effective alternatives now.

Thioridazine (Mellaril)

Thioridazine was commonly used as a well-tolerated, sedating medication, often given in small doses to people who did not have a psychotic illness. Recently, it was shown to cause a substantial increase in the QTc interval (the time that it takes the heart to repolarize and prepare for its next contraction). Many medications including ziprasidone (Geodon) cause this increase in the QTc interval, but thioridazine causes this much more than most other medications still on the market. While ziprasidone is fairly safe, thioridazine has at least a moderate risk for causing sudden death. As a result, thioridazine is now used only rarely, almost entirely in people who have been on it for years and do not want to switch despite the risk.

Side Effects. It is used in the same dose as chlorpromazine, except that it should never be used above 800 mg/day and only rarely above 400 mg/day because of its potential to damage the retina, causing permanent blindness. Thioridazine is a sedating medication that seems to be tolerated better than chlorpromazine and has fewer depressant side effects.

Specifics of Use. Thioridazine is more dangerous than other available medications and is now rarely used. Because it is sedating, it is often given once a day before bed. Other people use it in small doses during the day to calm down. It has historically been used in low doses, 10 to 50 mg, to calm people who are agitated and developmentally delayed or demented or who have a personality disorder. In a higher dose, usually around 400 mg/day, it is also effective in people with schizophrenia. In general, an EKG should be obtained before starting thioridazine, especially in anyone who is older, on other medications that can affect the heart, or has a known heart disease.

Fluphenazine (Prolixin)

Traditional dose range is 2–40 mg/day, although recent data suggest that the lower end of the range should be used in most cases. This medication is roughly 50 times as potent as chlorpromazine, and is a high-potency, low-dose, "least-sedating" phenothiazine. It can be given by mouth or by short-acting injection (Prolixin hydrochloride) or as a long-acting esterified injectable form that lasts for over two weeks called fluphenazine decanoate (Prolixin Decanoate).

Haloperidol (Haldol)

The dose range is 1–40 mg/day, although current research suggests that 5 mg/day is an effective dose for many people with schizophrenia. Haloperidol is chemically a butyrophenome rather than a phenothiazine. Despite this difference in its chemistry, it seems to work identically to other phenothiazine medications. It is a very high-potency antipsychotic, and, like Prolixin, it is roughly 50 times as potent as chlorpromazine. Twenty mg/day of haloperidol is roughly equivalent to 1,000 mg of chlorpromazine. It also comes in a long-acting injection called haloperidol decanoate (Haldol Decanoate) that can be given once a month.

Molindone (Moban)

The dosage is 20–225 mg/day. In most ways, molindone is similar to the phenothiazines, except that it may cause less weight gain than other antipsychotics. It is commonly used as a backup for people who have not responded well to other medications.

Thiothixene (Navane)

The dosage is 5–60 mg/day. Thiothixene is roughly 25 times as potent as chlorpromazine. It is chemically similar to chlorpromazine but is much less sedating and is advertised as being well-tolerated and having few side effects. It has somewhat less EPS effects than the higher potency medications such as haloperidol.

LONG-ACTING INJECTIONS

Long-acting injections of antipsychotic medications have traditionally been used when there is concern that someone would not take the medication on his or her own, or when there is concern that oral medications are not being efficiently absorbed. At this moment, only fluphenazine (Prolixin) and haloperidol (Haldol) are available in the United States in a long-acting injectable preparation. Fluphenazine and haloperidol deconoate work by combining the active medication with decanoic acid—a large fatty acid molecule. When this is injected, it takes the body some time to break the bond between the active medication and this larger molecule, and the active medication is therefore released gradually over several weeks. Unfortunately, these deconoate injections can cause irritation at the injection site, and at times can leave small hardened areas at the site (called "knots"). Both have all of the side effects of the other traditional antipsychotic medications, and so they are used as something of a last resort. It is expected that risperidone, now only available as a pill or liquid, will be available as a long-acting injection in the near future. Long-acting injections of some of the other atypical antipsychotic medications are likely to follow over the next few years. The role of long-acting injections is likely to increase once the atypical antipsychotics are available in this form.

Some people prefer receiving an injection every two to four weeks to taking a pill daily. The long-acting injection means that they do not have to remember to take a pill every day, and do not have to organize their life around the taking of medication. For others, taking a pill every day is a daily reminder that they have an illness. For other people, every pill requires a struggle with their own ambivalence over the medication. For still others, an injectable medication can decrease the "hassle" that sometimes occurs between consumer and family or consumer and staff, over whether the medication is really taken. Too often, too much attention is focused on whether the person has been taking his or her prescribed medication; the use of a long-acting injection can change the focus on medication to other parts of the person's life. A person who requires fluphenazine or haloperidol decanoate injections after discharge should probably be started on the short-acting form of the same medication as soon as possible so that side effects can be assessed.

Dose equivalency between oral medication and long-acting injection is highly variable from client to client. As a rough rule of thumb, 10 mg/day of oral Prolixin is equivalent to a 12.5 mg (½ cc) injection of Prolixin Decanoate every two weeks. Ten mg/day of oral Haldol is roughly equivalent to a 100 mg injection of Haldol Decanoate every four weeks (i.e., ten times the daily oral dose, given by injection every month). There is some difference between the two medications' pharmacokinetic properties (the way drugs are absorbed and metabolized or, in other words, the speed of onset and how long they remain in the body). With Prolixin Decanoate, the client tends to establish an effective serum level of medication within a day or two. With Haldol Decanoate, there is a gradual, smoother uptake of medication, and it may take several weeks or more to get an effective serum level.

Because of this slow uptake, it is often useful to start Haldol Decanoate with a higher "loading dose" by giving more medication during the first two months and then decreasing to a baseline dose. A person on 10 mg/day of oral Haldol could be given 200 mg of Haldol Decanoate through several injections during the first two months, and then slowly given decreasing amounts until a baseline dose of 100 mg/month was reached. Prolixin has the advantage of working faster after a single injection but has the disadvantage of having more side effects a few days after each injection.

Haldol Decanoate stays in the body longer than the Prolixin. Haldol Decanoate's half-life is approximately 21 days, which means that it would take five times that, or more than 100 days, for any dose change to completely equilibrate at a new blood level. Most people do well with a Haldol Decanoate injection once a month. Prolixin Decanoate's half-life is approximately 14 days, which means that injections are typically given every two weeks and that it would take 40–60 days for any dose change to equilibrate at a new blood level.

Risperidone Long-Acting Injections

A risperidone long-acting injection is expected to be available in early 2003. It would be called Risperdal long-acting microsphere (Risperdal Consta). This new injection works through a very different mechanism from that of the older long-acting medications. Instead of combining the active medication with a deconoate molecule, it encapsulates the risperidone in a polymer, making what is called a "microsphere" or microscopically small capsule. This breaks apart over three to six weeks, releasing the active medication. The material making up this capsule completely breaks down into lactic acid and other natural products, so that nothing remains behind to cause knots.

At this time, relatively few people have used Risperidone Consta. While it seems very promising, we will have more information as more people try it. Initial studies suggest that there is much less injection site pain than with the older injections. It also seems as though the slow release may have some clinical advantages. (1) Since the release is slow, the peak blood levels of the medication are lower than with pills, which may cause fewer side effects. (2) Because of the steady, low blood levels, the metabolism of the medication appears to be a bit different than with pills, allowing lower doses to be effective and again decreasing side effects. (3) Even people who are relatively consistent with their medication tend to miss some doses; as mentioned above, using long-acting injections avoids the attention focused on daily doses. Again, the consistency of action of long-lasting injections will allow some people to function much better than with pills.

Because of the nature of the microspheres, the injections need to be given every two weeks. It is unlikely that people will be able to vary the injection frequency as they often do with haloperidol or fluphenazine. There is also very little release at the time the first injection is given, so that there is essentially no active medication for the three weeks after the first injection. Because of the nature of the microspheres, all of the medication is out of the person's body seven or eight weeks after the last injection, even if they had been taking the injections for some time. If someone had been on either of the older medications, it could take many months for the medication to be completely gone after the injections were stopped. Although this long period of residual action was sometimes useful if someone stopped his or her medication, it raised concerns about ongoing side effects if someone had a problem with the medication.

It appears that most people will need between 25 and 50 mg every two weeks. While the 25 mg dose provides a serum level roughly equivalent to 2 mg of oral risperidone a day, for many people it appears to be a much more effective dose than this serum level would suggest.

SIDE EFFECTS FOR ALL ANTIPSYCHOTIC MEDICATIONS

Side effects of the antipsychotic medications can be divided into four broad categories. The first is extrapyramidal, or muscle-related, side effects. The second group includes common, non-muscle-related side effects that are uncomfortable but not life-threatening. The third covers those side effects that are rare, dangerous, and can lead to permanent difficulties. The fourth includes weight gain and diabetes; both are enough of a problem with the atypical antipsychotic medications that they rate their own category.

Extrapyramidal Effects

Pyramidal cells are nerve cells in the brain that are involved in the control of voluntary muscle movements. Extrapyramidal refers to the part of the central nervous system concerned with control and coordination of muscle movements not part of the main pyramidal tracts (hence the term extrapyramidal). These are common and uncomfortable but not dangerous complications of antipsychotic drug use. They can increase the discomfort of many people and frequently prompt people to refuse to take medications. They are usually treatable, and, except for tardive dyskinesia, all disappear when drugs are discontinued. Tardive dyskinesia has no reliable treatment and may be permanent even after antipsychotic medications are stopped.

Extrapyramidal side effects are much less frequent with the atypical antipsychotic medications, including clozapine, risperidone, olanzapine, quetiapine, and ziprasidone. In addition, the atypical antipsychotic medications appear less likely to cause tardive dyskinesia. Less likely is not the same as zero. The newer medications can cause extrapyramidal side effects, and they can cause tardive dyskinesia.

Dystonia symptoms include sudden, often dramatic, spasms of muscles of head, neck, lips, and tongue. Tilted head, slurred speech, or eyes deviated up or to one side are also common. Dystonias can be very frightening and at times are dismissed as bizarre behavior rather than recognized as a drug side effect. Dystonias usually occur hours or days after the medication is started or the dose is increased. They are easily treated with anticholinergic drugs like benztropine (Cogentin) at 1–2 mg by mouth or intramuscular injection, or diphenhydramine (Benadryl) at 25 mg by intramuscular injection for rapid relief. Dystonias are very rare with atypical antipsychotics.

Pseudoparkinsonism usually consists of muscular rigidity, mask-like face, and stiff walk with loss of normal arm swing and a shuffling gait. These people often have a coarse, 3 per/ sec tremor that is worse at rest than with activity. Pseudoparkinsonism usually begins after three weeks of treatment. Parkinson-type muscle rigidity, at least to the extent that it is grossly obvious, is rare with the atypical antipsychotics.

Akathisia is a late-appearing side effect that usually occurs 5–14 days after beginning medication. It is characterized by constant pacing, moving of hands or feet, and a feeling of nervousness. People can often distinguish this motor restlessness from anxiety and may say things like "it feels like my motor is running all of the time." *Akathisia is a common, very uncomfortable, and often unrecognized side effect that is one of the frequent reasons that people discontinue their medication.* Akathisia often becomes more severe if the person is already anxious and can become somewhat better if the person can relax. This can be very confusing since akathisia is easily confused with anxiety in the first place. Akathisia can also be confused with an exacerbation of the underlying psychosis. Some people find that caffeine makes it worse.

While akathisia is less common with the atypical than with the traditional medications, it is not unusual especially when the dose of the medication is raised to high levels. Risperidone is most likely to cause akathisia, especially as the dose is increased above 4 or 6 mg/day. Quetiapine and clozapine are least likely to cause it. There is little information about ziprasidone although there is reason to believe that it may be a bit like risperidone where akathisia is more of a problem as the dose is increased.

Akathisia is very uncomfortable and often very difficult to treat. It is one of the more common reasons that people discontinue antipsychotic medications and has even been cited as a cause of suicide. Reducing the dose of the antipsychotic medication is the first thing that should be considered, but uncomfortable symptoms may persist. Akathisia is often unresponsive to anticholinergic medications. Beta-blocking medications such as propranolol (Inderal) are often effective in treating akathisia. Anxiolytics (minor tranquilizers) such as diazepam (Valium) can also be very helpful with akathisia that is unresponsive to other treatment.

Akinesia is frequently overlooked and can be difficult to distinguish from the psychiatric illness for which the drug is being prescribed. It is manifested by loss of spontaneity in facial expression or gesturing, being "slowed up," or shuffling. More subtle but still uncomfortable parts of this syndrome are seen in decreased social spontaneity, diminished conversation, apathy, and disinclination to initiate normal activity. Akinesia is partially treatable with anticholinergic medication, but it is often treatment resistant and can be an ongoing clinical problem.

Tardive dyskinesia appears late, usually after years of medication use, and seems to be related to total lifetime dose of medication. Once it appears in full-blown syndrome, *it can be permanent.* It is estimated to affect 20–30% of people chronically using antipsychotic medications and appears more frequently in women, the elderly, and people with a diagnosis other than schizophrenia. It can be stopped by early recognition and discontinuation of the antipsychotic medication. Some studies have suggested that abnormally frequent eye-blinking may be an early sign of tardive dyskinesia in some people. In other people, the first sign is a writhing motion of the tongue. If the medication is continued, this can progress to rhythmic, disfiguring distortion of the mouth or face. Other parts of the body can also be involved. There are a number of common scales, including the AIMS (abnormal involuntary movement scale), that allow clinicians to monitor and track early symptoms of tardive dyskinesia.

Some people who get very mild tardive dyskinesia find that it never worsens, even if they stay on antipsychotic medications. In other people it can progress fairly rapidly over a period of months to become a very disfiguring and incapacitating movement disorder. It is impossible to predict who is at risk for progression to the severe form and who is not. As more people are treated with antipsychotic agents for longer periods of time, tardive dyskinesia is likely to become increasingly problematic.

There is a debate currently under way about the risk of tardive dyskinesia with the atypical antipsychotic medications. It is certainly substantially less than with the traditional medications, but it is unclear if the risk of tardive dyskinesia is around

2-3% of people taking the atypical medications, or if the risk is even much lower.

Benztropine (Cogentin) and other anticholinergic drugs can usually control most EPS effects, but they often make tardive dyskinesia worse rather than better. As with other EPS effects, symptoms of tardive dyskinesia typically disappear with sleep and are made worse by increased anxiety. Similarly, caffeine often makes symptoms worse, although this varies from one client to another. There is some suggestion that vitamin E may decrease the chance of developing tardive dyskinesia and may be partially helpful in its treatment.

Common, Non-Muscle-Related Side Effects

Toxic side effects can affect anyone taking antipsychotic medications, at least to some extent. They are usually dose-related and sometimes can be controlled by changing doses, taking most of the dose at night, or switching medications. Symptoms include drowsiness or feeling "drugged," sluggish, and unmotivated. They are much less of a problem with the atypicals than with older medications. Drug-induced or drug-potentiated depressions also may occur.

Psychotoxic effects include depression, depersonalization, dysphoria, akinesia, confusion, and somatic delusion. *Remember, antipsychotic drugs can make things worse as well as better.* These side effects, which are connected to the feeling of being "drugged," all seem to be much less of a problem with atypical antipsychotic medications.

Anticholinergic side effects. Anticholinergic refers to medications that block the receptors of the neurotransmitter acetylcholine. While most antipsychotic medications have at least some anticholinergic activity, it is not usually a problem with the atypical antipsychotics except for clozapine, which has a lot of anticholinergic activity. Most anticholinergic side effects come from the medications used to treat muscle side effects, such as benztropine (Cogentin) or trihexphenidyl (Artane). Some of the antihistamines, such as benadryl, are also very anticholinergic. The most common anticholinergic side effects include dry mouth, blurred vision, and constipation. Anticholinergic medications block sweating and can interfere with temperature regulation, leaving the person much more susceptible to heat stroke. They can make it difficult to loosen the muscles controlling the sphincter of the bladder, causing urinary retention (especially in older men). In overdoses, anticholinergic medications can cause a delirium that can look something like an increase in the person's psychosis. All anticholinergic medications can interfere with memory, especially in the elderly or with people whose memory is already impaired from some other problem.

Alpha-adrenergic side effects. Adrenaline works on two different kinds of nerve receptors: alpha and beta. Medications that block the alpha-receptors can cause orthostatic hypotension (sudden drop in blood pressure when the client suddenly stands up), which can cause some transient dizziness and can cause the client to fall down. Broken bones in older people are a frequent problem made worse by alpha-adrenergic medications. Alpha-adrenergic effects are worse with low-potency drugs like Thorazine and Mellaril. Among the atypicals, effects are worse with clozapine and risperidone.

Medications that block the D_2 receptor all cause an increase in prolactin, a sex-related hormone that can cause breast enlargement and secretion of breast liquid from both men and women. Prolactin elevation also interferes with menstrual periods in women, seems related to decreased sex drive, and, over long periods of time, may possibly be connected to a loss of bone calcium leading to increased risk of osteoporosis. All the traditional antipsychotic medications increase prolactin, as does risperidone (Risperdal). Other atypicals do not seem to cause significant prolactin elevation.

Photosensitivity reactions happen when the skin becomes very sensitive to sunlight. Again, Thorazine is the most common drug to cause this effect.

Rare, but Serious and Potentially Permanent, Side Effects

Blood dyscrasias. Many people put on antipsychotic medication have a partial block on the production of certain blood elements, usually white cells and platelets. This is usually of no clinical significance and within a few days the system is back to normal. Occasionally, the white blood count continues to decrease slowly (leukopenia) in a dose-related reaction without other symptoms. This decrease must be monitored closely, and sometimes switching to a different medication is necessary. If this temporary block is relatively complete and the system does not return to normal, the rapid decrease in white cells and/or platelets quickly becomes life-threatening. Such a complete block is very rare but can be more common with low-potency, high-dose drugs (Thorazine and Mellaril). It is *much* more common with clozapine (Clozaril).

People are at highest risk for a block in making white blood cells (agranulocytosis) in the first two to four months after starting a new medication. Symptoms include weakness, high fever, chills, and a sore throat. *A physician should be called and a CBC (complete blood count) ordered immediately if someone develops a high fever or chills within weeks of starting a new medication.* The outcome depends on how rapidly a diagnosis is made. If the client has a blood dyscrasia, all medication must be stopped immediately.

Neuroleptic malignant syndrome (NMS) usually occurs within a few weeks of starting an antipsychotic medication and is marked by a very high temperature and muscle stiffness. Other early signs include confusion, increased pulse, and increased blood pressure. People can easily die from hyperthermia (body temperature above 105°) if not rapidly and vigorously treated. *Any client taking an antipsychotic medication who complains of an increased temperature and muscular rigidity should be evaluated for NMS.*

Temperature regulation. All antipsychotic medications can interfere with a person's normal temperature-regulation mechanisms in hot weather. During the 1995 heat wave in Wisconsin, a number of people taking these medications died, including several young men who would not normally be considered at risk for fatal heatstroke.

People on antipsychotic medications, especially low-potency medications such as clozapine and chlorpromazine (Thorazine), are much more likely to suffer a potentially fatal heatstroke. People taking these medications should have air conditioners or fans or have a cool place to go to if their living accommodations become too hot. They should also drink fluids to avoid becoming dehydrated.

Cardiovascular effects. Many medications slightly increase the time it takes for electrical impulses to spread through the heart. They also increase the time required for the heart to "repolarize," or reset, after the last heartbeat in preparation for its next beat. This is called the QT interval, the time from the beginning of the "Q" wave to the end of the "T" wave on and EKG. The QTc interval is the QT interval corrected for heart rate. Increases in the QTc interval have been associated with sudden death. The risk increases as the QTc interval goes above 450 msec (milliseconds), and becomes significant above 500 msec.

Thioridazine (Mellaril) causes the biggest change of QTc interval. This increase is large enough that thioridazine should be used with caution. Ziprasidone also causes an increase in the QTc interval, but it is a much smaller increase than with thioridazine. The risk from QTc prolongation with ziprasidone seems fairly small. An EKG is not needed in otherwise healthy people. An EKG is probably indicated before starting ziprasidone in someone who is older, has a known heart disease, or is taking other medications that significantly increase QTc interval. Note that many medications increase QTc to a slight extent, but this long list of common medications would not prompt the need for an EKG.

Clozapine has also been associated with myocarditis, an inflammation of the heart. The FDA has recently issued a warning about this risk. There have been 30 reported cases, including 17 fatalities, in the United States. Since slightly over 200,000 people have taken clozapine, often for many years, this gives a fatality rate of 2.8 per 100,000 patient-years on the medication. The possibility of myocarditis should be considered for anyone taking clozapine who complains of unexpected fatigue, shortness of breath, rapid pulse, fever, or chest pain. It is important to consider the possibility of mycarditis since some of these symptoms, such as tiredness and rapid pulse, are common for many people taking clozapine.

Eye problems. Blurred vision is a common, reversible side effect from all of these medications, especially the high-dose medications like chlorpromazine and clozapine. This is an "anticholinergic" side effect and is made worse by other anticholinergic medications, including medications used for extrapyramidal side effects like benztropine or by antidepressants like amitriptyline. The blurred vision goes away when the medication is discontinued.

Lens opacities (cataracts) are a rare but more serious side effect, especially of long-term chlorpromazine and possibly quetiapine use. Thioridazine (Mellaril) has been reported to cause deposition of the pigments in the retina that can lead to blindness. This is rare in people taking less than 800 mg/day for a lengthy period of time.

Seizures. All of these medications lower the seizure threshold. Seizures are rare in people taking these medications but are something to consider, especially with people who already have difficulty controlling epilepsy. Some of these medications, such as clozapine, are much more likely to cause seizures than other antipsychotic medications, especially when used in higher doses. Seizures are rarely dangerous (unless the person happens to be driving at the time), but they are frightening to both the client and observers.

Weight Gain and Diabetes

Weight gain. All of the antipsychotic medications (with the exception of ziprasidone) are associated with weight gain. Weight gain is most likely with olanzapine and clozapine, intermediate with risperidone, less with haloperidol and least with ziprasidone. Not everyone on these medications gains weight, but it is common. The exact cause of the weight gain is unclear, but it seems related to carbohydrate craving. People on these medications often feel hungrier. Weight gain is a problem for people's self-image and general sense of well-being. It is also a significant medical problem. Obesity is related to a range of medical problems including heart disease and diabetes.

Diabetes. Diabetes is a common and serious medical illness. It is associated with blindness, heart disease, kidney problems, and stroke. Diabetes is more common in people with schizophrenia than in the general population. It is also much more common in people who are overweight. Many people with schizophrenia are overweight from a variety of factors, including poor diet, inactivity, less exercise, and perhaps factors related to schizophrenia itself. The significant weight gain associated with some of the atypical antipsychotic medications is certainly a factor in the increased frequency of diabetes observed among people with schizophrenia.

In addition to the diabetes associated with weight gain, there is growing concern that the atypical antipsychotic medications, especially clozapine and olanzapine, can cause diabetes even in the absence of weight gain. The medications seem to cause direct changes in how the body handles glucose and insulin.

Interactions with Street Drugs

Many people taking antipsychotic medications also abuse alcohol or street drugs. Alcohol and other sedating medications can increase the sedative side effects of the antipsychotic medications. Many illicit drugs also have anticholinergic effects that can increase the anticholinergic side effects of the prescribed medications. Finally, many people with mental illnesses are particularly susceptible to the paranoia or psychotic effects obtained from many illicit drugs. Despite this increased risk from the illicit drugs themselves, there are few medically dangerous interactions between normal doses of alcohol or illicit drugs and normally prescribed levels of antipsychotic medications.

Use during Pregnancy

It cannot be proven that any medication is absolutely safe during pregnancy. These drugs do cross the placenta, but there is no evidence that antipsychotic medications increase the risk of birth defects. While all pregnant women should, as a general rule, take as few medications as possible, pregnancy should not be a reason to completely avoid antipsychotic drug use. The stress of psychosis is also potentially damaging to the fetus, and the various risks must be weighed against each other. These drugs will also appear in breast milk. Again, while there is no absolute contraindication, it is probably safer for mothers taking these medications not to breast feed their babies.

TABLE 5. *Side Effects and Potency of Antipsychotic Medications*

	Dose Equivalent to 100 mg of Chlorpromazine	Sedation	Anticholinergic Side Effects	EPSE	Orthostatic Hypotension
chlorpromazine (Thorazine)	100 mg	+++	++	++	+++
clozapine (Clozaril)	50 mg	+++	+++	+/−	+++
fluphenazine (Prolixin)	2 mg	+	+	+++	+
haloperidol (Haldol)	2 mg	+	+	+++	+
loxapine (Loxitane)	10 mg	++	+	+++	++
mesoridazine (Serentil)	50 mg	+++	+++	+	++
molindone (Moban)	10 mg	+	+	+++	+
olanzapine (Zyprexa)	5 mg	++	+	+/−	+
perphenazine (Trilafon)	8 mg	+	+	+++	+
prochlorperazine (Compazine)	15 mg	++	+	+++	+
risperidone (Risperdal)	2 mg	+	+	+	+
thioridazine (Mellaril)	100 mg	+++	+++	+	+++
thiothixene (Navane)	4 mg	+	+	+++	+
trifluoperazine (Stelazine)	5 mg	+	+	+++	+

Key: +Mild ++Moderate +++Severe +/−Minimal
Adapted from *Drug Facts and Comparisons*, 1997, St. Louis, MO: Facts and Comparisons.

TABLE 6. *Detailed Side Effect Profile of Atypical Antipsychotic Medications*

	Typical Antipsychotic	Clozapine	Risperidone	Olanzapine	Quetiapine	Ziprasidone
Agitation	+ to ++	–	+	+	+/–	++
Agranulocytosis	rare	+++	rare	rare	rare	rare
Anticholinergic effects	+ to +++	+++	+/–	++	+	+
Dose-related EPS effects increase	yes	no	yes	yes	no	yes
EPS effects	+ to +++	–	+	–	–	+
Liver enzyme abnormalities	+	+	–	+	+	+
Nausea/heartburn	+	++	+/–	+	–	++
Orthostatic hypotension	+ to +++	+++	++	+	++	++
Prolactin increase	+++	–	+++	+/–	+/–	–
Sedation	++ to +++	+++	+	++	+++	– to +
Seizures	+	+++	+	+	+	+
Tardive dyskinesia	+++	rare	+	+	rare	+
Weight gain	+	+++	++	+++	++	–

Key: +Mild ++Moderate +++Severe +/–Minimal –None

TABLE 7. *Common Side Effects of Medications Used to Treat Schizophrenia*

Side Effect	Description	May be Confused with . . .
Akathisia	• Feeling restless or jittery • Needing to fidget, stand up, or pace around	• Anxiety • Psychotic symptoms • Cocaine intoxication • Alcohol withdrawal
Akinesia	• Feeling slowed-down • Losing normal spontaneity • No mental energy ("I feel like a zombie")	• Negative symptoms of schizophrenia • Depression
Anticholinergic effects (physical)	• Dry mouth • Blurry vision • Trouble urinating • Constipation	• None
Anticholinergic effects (mental)	• Memory difficulties • Confusion (feeling "spacy") • Visual hallucinations	• Symptoms of schizophrenia • Drug intoxication • Depression
Dystonia	• Sudden muscle spasm or charley horse (usually happens when antipsychotic medication is started or dose is raised; most common with high-potency traditional antipsychotics)	• Strange movements that occur during psychotic episodes by stress and that can be mistaken for hysterical reactions or malingering
Sexual and menstrual difficulties	• Loss of sexual desire • Loss of erection or ejaculation • Cessation of menses	• Low sex drive can also be due to schizophrenia or depression • Menstrual irregularities often caused by medications and rarely directly caused by schizophrenia
Tardive dyskinesia	• Writhing movements of mouth, tongue, or hands, or any other repetitive movements	• Tremor • Transient movements associated with antipsychotic dose reductions • Spontaneous movements seen in people with schizophrenia even without medication exposure

(continued)

TABLE 7. *Continued*

Side Effect	Description	May be Confused with . . .
Tremor	• Shaking of hands or other parts of body	
Weight gain	• Common with all antipsy-chotics, but worse with atypical antipsychotics (with the exception of ziprasidone)	• Associated with inactivity and poor diet, but is also a direct effect of medication. Do not blame person for weight gain.

4

Antidepressant Medications

Antidepressant medications can be divided into four large classes. They are (1) the new generation of antidepressants that work either through the serotonin or norepinephrine system, including the selective serotonin reuptake inhibitors (SSRIs), such as fluoxetine (Prozac) and sertraline (Zoloft), and a variety of other antidepressants that work through the same neurotransmitter systems by different mechanisms, (2) antidepressants that have important activity in the dopamine system, e.g., bupropion (Wellbutrin), (3) tricyclic antidepressants, e.g., desipramine (Norpramin) and nortriptyline (Pamelor), and (4) the monoamine oxidase inhibitors (MAOIs), e.g., phenelzine (Nardil) and tranylcypromine (Parnate).

Medications within any one class are more similar to each other than they are different, and while there are some important differences within a class, they are primarily differences in side effects. As with the antipsychotic medications, some people will respond much better to one medication than to another, even if the medications are similar and from the same class. Someone who does not respond to an SSRI may respond well to another SSRI.

The older generation of antidepressants had so many side effects and made people feel so drugged that people discontinued them as rapidly as possible. The newer antidepressants are much easier to live with. People who have had a single depressive episode can often discontinue antidepressant medication after 6–12 months; while they may be at risk for another period of depression later in their lives, they are likely to do well for years without medication. People with multiple episodes of depression, or who have a chronic depression may do better if they stay on antidepressant medication for a long period of time. This is an individual decision. A large number of people continue on antidepressant medications indefinitely because they feel that life is better when they take them. At times, antidepressant medications seem to stop working. This "poop out" effect is not uncommon. Raising the dose of the medication or switching to another antidepressant is usually effective.

Mania and Rapid Cycling. All effective antidepressants can precipitate mania in people who are susceptible. Antidepressants can also make rapid cycling worse. There are some people who alternate between being depressed and either hypomanic or full manic. All antidepressants can increase the frequency and the intensity of these cycles.

Before starting any antidepressant, obtain a medical history. The best antidepressant to start with is one that worked in the past for either that person or someone in his or her immediate family. Always obtain a history of medical illness and the list of medications including herbs and over-the-counter medications that the person is already taking.

Withdrawal Effects. All of the antidepressants can cause withdrawal symptoms. While withdrawal is not medically dangerous, it can cause people to feel more depressed, irritable, develop flu-like symptoms and have trouble sleeping. A slow decrease off of antidepressants rather than abruptly stopping them will almost always keep symptoms from occurring.

Note on Terminology. Adrenalin and epinephrine are the same chemical, despite having different names. Similarly, noradrenalin and norepinephrine are different names for the same chemical. The adrenaline system is often called the adrenergic system. Serotonin is chemically described as 5-hydroxy-tryptamine or 5-HT. 5-HT is a common abbreviation for serotonin. Most antidepressants work through either the adrenergic or serotonergic system, or a combination of the two.

INDICATIONS FOR USE OF ANTIDEPRESSANTS

Depression

It is often difficult to predict which depressed person will respond to antidepressant medications and which person will not. People who are more likely to respond to medication may experience weight loss, waking in the early morning, feeling worse in the morning but better as the day goes on, or suffering from depressions lacking a major reactive component (that is, there is no obvious reason why they are depressed). A pervasive sense of anhedonia (when things the person used to enjoy are no longer fun) and a sense of hopelessness are other classic characteristics of depressed people who respond to antidepressant medications. Many of these people have a family member who is depressed, alcoholic, or has made suicide attempts.

There are a number of different kinds of "depression" in the *Diagnostic and Statistical Manual of Mental Disorders* (*DSM-IV*). Major depression is severe and interferes with the person's ability to function. Dysthymia is a persistent, less intense depression that can stay with the person for years. While major depression is more dramatic, dysthymia can cause people to feel miserable, interfere with their ability to feel pleasure, and it can cause major problems in relationships. Both types are treatable. Treatment in most cases involves psychotherapy with either an interpersonal or cognitive-behavioral approach and medication. It often makes sense for someone with dysthymia to start with psychotherapy, but antidepressant medication should be considered if the depression continues. Antidepressant medications seem ineffective for people going through a typical grief reaction or for a depression that seems primarily reactive to negative life events, although if a person gets "stuck" in grieving an antidepressant may be indicated.

Most people with depression do very well with just one antidepressant and do not need a combination of different medications. At times, however, combining antidepressant medications makes sense. The goal is not just to decrease the depression, but to get the person completely over it. At times, combinations of medication are needed to accomplish this.

At times, antidepressants are combined with other kinds of medications. People who are agitated or have major sleep problems may respond faster if given an antianxiety medication, such as diazepam (Valium), for a few days at the beginning of treatment, in addition to an antidepressant. Some people with a very agitated depression, especially if they have psychotic symptoms, initially respond better to a combination of an antipsychotic medication and an antidepressant. People with a delusional depression initially respond much better to antipsychotic and antidepressant medications than to antidepressants alone. Antidepressant medications can be used with antipsychotics, common sleeping pills, or electroconvulsive therapy (ECT). Antidepressants are useful in combination with lithium or other mood stabilizers in people who are in the depressed phase of a manic-depressive illness.

Anxiety Disorders

These medications are called "antidepressants" because they were first used to treat depression. They are, however, effective for a number of other conditions, and they just as easily could have been called "antipanic" medications. Most antidepressants—with the exception of bupropion (Wellbutrin)—are useful for anxiety disorders, whether or not the person is depressed.

We used to talk about anxiety as though it were a single disorder. There is increasing agreement that there are a number of different anxiety disorders, each with their own biology and each responding somewhat differently to treatment. All of them respond to antidepressants, but not all of them respond to the traditional Valium-type antianxiety medications. The current diagnostic system lists five different anxiety disorders: panic, obsessive-compulsive disorder (OCD), generalized anxiety disorder (GAD), social phobia, and posttraumatic stress disorder (PTSD).

Panic. Panic is very intense, very brief periods of extreme anxiety. People often feel that they are dying or having a heart attack. Panic attacks often occur when the person is relaxed, without any apparent stresses. Often, people with ongoing panic develop a fear of being in places where they may be trapped. As a result, they avoid crowded places like shopping centers or open areas where they cannot return home rapidly. This fear of being outside is called agoraphobia. Panic can be so severe and frequent as to cause major problems in people's lives. It can be so upsetting that it can make some people suicidal. Almost all of the antidepressants (except bupropion [Wellbutrin]) are effective for treating panic. Because they are less addicting and less sedating than the benzodiazepines, they have become the "first-line" medications for panic.

Obsessive-Compulsive Disorder (OCD). Strongly serotonergic medications, especially the SSRIs and clomipramine, are extremely helpful with many people who have this often disabling disorder. OCD sometimes requires a higher dose of medication than depression does. For example, 20 mg of fluoxetine (Prozac) is generally an effective dose for most people with depression and most people with OCD. Some people with OCD may require 60–80 mg/day. All of the SSRI medications seem equally effective for OCD, although there is less research for some than others.

Clomipramine (Anafranil) sometimes works for people with OCD who do not respond to the SSRIs. I do not use it as my first medication of choice because it has many more side effects than the SSRIs. Clomipramine is sedating and causes weight gain, dry mouth, and constipation, and it is lethal when taken as an overdose. However, it sometimes helps with OCD when other medications are ineffective.

Typically, one starts clomipramine at 25 mg/day and then increases the dose to 150 mg/day. A typical dose range is 150–250 mg/day.

Generalized Anxiety Disorder (GAD). Until recently, it was thought that antidepressants were generally ineffective for GAD. A number of research studies (and clinical experience) suggests that most antidepressants (except bupropion [Wellbutrin]) are useful for GAD. Unlike a benzodiazepine that starts working right away, most people need to take an antidepressant regularly for several weeks before it begins to be effective. It has less of an initial "kick" than a benzodiazepine, so people may not feel that they are as effective. Benzodiazepines are safe and effective when prescribed and taken appropriately, but the antidepressants are less addicting and for the most part less sedating. They may also cause fewer cognitive problems such as the memory problems that some people report with benzodiazepines.

Social Phobia. People with social phobia can become so fearful of how other people may judge them that they almost become recluses. This is a common condition and can interfere with all areas of a person's life. A number of different medications including most of the antidepressants can decrease the intensity of the fear.

Posttraumatic Stress Disorder (PTSD). Antidepressants are commonly used to decrease the depression commonly associated with PTSD and are often combined with other medications to treat the various symptoms of startle, intrusive nightmares, and overarousal that are common symptoms.

Bulimia

Most of the antidepressants (including all of the tricyclics and SSRIs) are helpful for at least some people with bulimia, whether they are depressed or not. These medications can decrease the frequency and severity of the bingeing and help people with bulimia to establish more control over their own eating.

Cocaine Craving and Depression

It has been proposed that antidepressants may help people cope with symptoms of cocaine withdrawal. Desipramine has been most frequently studied, but other antidepressants are also rumored to be effective for this purpose. Recent data suggest that antidepressants can treat the postwithdrawal depression that is very common in heavy, habitual users, but there is much less support for the idea that these medications help with cocaine cravings or withdrawal. As is the case with treating depression, there is often a delay of several weeks between starting the medication and seeing a positive response.

Smoking Cessation

Bupropion, in combination with a nicotine patch and a smoking cessation program, seems effective in helping motivated people quit smoking. This is specific to bupropion. Other antidepressants do not appear effective in decreasing smoking. The bupropion should be started 7–10 days before the designated "stop smoking" day, while the nicotine patch is started when the cigarettes are stopped. Generally, a normal antidepressant dose is used. Bupropion can be started at 100 mg twice a day for three days and then increased to 150 mg twice a day. Bupropion is marketed under the name Wellbutrin when used as an antidepressant and as Zyban when used as part of a smoking cessation program. They are exactly the same medication.

Other Conditions for Which Antidepressants Are Useful

Antidepressants are also useful for a variety of other conditions. They can increase the effectiveness of some pain medications and are used to treat some migraine-type headaches. Neurologists prescribe them regularly. They can treat a variety of what are called "stage-four sleep disorders," which include night terrors and enuresis in children. Finally, they can be very helpful for fibromyalgia symptoms.

TYPES OF ANTIDEPRESSANTS

Medications that Work Selectively through the Serotonin and/or Norepinephrine System

Almost all of the currently available antidepressants—except bupropion (Wellbutrin)—work by influencing either norepinephrine or serotonin or both. The first generation antidepressants, the tricyclics and MAOIs, worked through these same systems but affected many other systems throughout the brain and the body, causing many side effects. The new antidepressants are much more selective, acting more precisely on the parts of the neurotransmitters that seem related to depression. This means that they are far safer and cause fewer side effects than the older medications. While the new medications may be more effective in treating anxiety disorders than the older medications, they do not appear any more effective in treating depression. They are, however, safer and easier to live with.

Selective Serotonin Reuptake Inhibitors (SSRIs)

The first of these new antidepressants selectively blocked the reuptake of serotonin. The selective serotonin reuptake inhibitors (SSRIs) include fluoxetine (Prozac), sertraline (Zoloft), and paroxetine (Paxil). Prozac was the first of these new antidepressants and was widely publicized as something of a "miracle drug." It was even featured on the cover of *Newsweek*. It has also been attacked by various groups for precipitating suicides, although data do not support this claim. The reality is that these new medications are not miracle drugs. For typical depression, they are no more effective than the older tricyclic-type antidepressants. Their major advantage is that they are much safer and are generally better tolerated than the older medications.

How They Work. A nerve cell communicates with the next cell by releasing a chemical called a neurotransmitter that activates receptors on the next cell. After this release, the neurotransmitter must be removed or deactivated before the cell receptors can become active again. There are two primary ways that this deactivation can occur. One is to break the neurotransmitter molecule into smaller, inactive pieces. The second is to literally suck the neurotransmitter back into the cell that just released it, so that it can be cleared from the space between the cells, repackaged, and used again. The selective reuptake inhibitors block this reuptake process, leaving a longer period of time for the serotonin to act on the receiving cell.

These new antidepressants are much more selective in blocking the targeted neurotransmitter than the older tricyclic-type antidepressants. While these medications do not appear to be more effective overall than the older medications, their selectivity decreases side effects. The serotonergic antidepressants may be particularly useful for people with anxiety disorders, especially obsessive-compulsive disorder (OCD).

The SSRIs are much more similar than they are different. For all practical purposes, if one of these medications is effective generally for a particular problem, all of the other medications in this same class will also work for the same problem. For reasons that are not exactly clear, people may respond to one of the medications in this group much better than another, so it is sometimes worth trying another one if the first does not work. While the side effects are all somewhat similar, there are some differences in the frequency of different side effects of different medications within this class.

Side Effects. SSRIs have different side-effect profiles than the older tricyclic antidepressants. As a group, they also are well tolerated with fewer side effects than the older antidepressants. Some people complain of nausea and headaches when a medication is first started, but this usually disappears in a few days or weeks. The SSRIs tend to be activating rather than sedating, and some people feel a sense of agitation or restlessness. The SSRIs can interfere with sleep in some people, while others report sedation and a sense of lethargy. Some people also feel "blunted" as though their emotional reaction is less than it was before starting medication. Motor restlessness (akathisia) is also sometimes a problem although it is rarer than with the antipsychotics.

SSRIs initially tend to cause less weight gain than older antidepressants. Roughly one out of four people on SSRIs gain weight over time, usually months after starting the medication. One study found an average weight gain of 4 pounds over 24 weeks. This did not seem related to an increase in appetite or food intake.

Sexual dysfunction, both difficulty having an orgasm and decreased libido, is a fairly common dose-related side effect of SSRIs. This is often a client's biggest complaint and often there is no good solution. The client can always switch to one of the other antidepressants with fewer sexual side effects. At times, adding bupropion (Wellbutrin) will reverse the sexual side effects caused by an SSRI. A long list of other medications have been used that may help some people, but none are reliable and all have their own side effects. Medications used to treat the sexual side effects of the SSRIs include cyproheptadine (Periactin), yohimbine (Yocon), amantadine (Symmetrel), and sildenafil (Viagra).

Suicide is always a risk for depressed people who are beginning to come out of their depression and become activated, but there is no evidence that SSRIs increase this risk. They are much less lethal after an overdose than tricyclic antidepressants and have fewer cardiac side effects.

Specifics of Use.

1. *Fluoxetine (Prozac).* Most depressed patients respond to a single 20 mg tablet a day, although elderly patients may not

tolerate this high a dose. People with OCD may do better with a higher dose—up to 60 mg/day. Fluoxetine has a half-life of more than 80 hours, which means that it remains in the body for weeks after someone stops taking it. This long half-life also means that some people can only take the medication two or three times a week rather than once a day.

There should be at least a five-week break between stopping fluoxetine and starting an MAOI. There is also some risk in immediately switching from fluoxetine and another antidepressant; a wash-out period of up to several weeks is recommended. This need for a medication-free period can be a major problem for people who want to switch but feel that they cannot tolerate the drug-free period. The other SSRIs have a shorter half-life and do not require as long a wash-out before another medication is started.

Fluoxetine is now available in generic form. This means it has gone from one of the more expensive antidepressants to one of the least expensive. The pharmaceutical company that developed fluoxetine has just marketed a long-acting, once-a-week version of the medication. This will be under a new patent and not available in generic form. In reality, the half-life of regular fluoxetine is so long that most people can take it once a week if this is preferred.

2. *Sertraline (Zoloft)* is typically started at 50 mg/day, and a typical dose is 50–200 mg/day. Its half-life is around 26 hours, but this varies considerably from one person to the next. All the SSRIs can raise the serum level of other medications, but Zoloft may do this a bit less than the others.

3. *Paroxetine (Paxil)*. A typical dose of paroxetine is 20 mg/day, with a range of 10–50 mg/day. It has been suggested that side effects of paroxetine include a lower incidence of nervousness and sleep problems than the other SSRIs. Paroxetine is also less expensive than other medications in this group. All the SSRIs can raise the serum level of many other medications, but paroxetine (along with sertraline) may do this a bit less than the others.

4. *Fluvoxamine (Luvox)* is an SSRI antidepressant that has been approved for use (along with clomipramine) for the treatment of OCD. It is usually started at 50 mg at bedtime, with a normal dose range of 100–300 mg/day. It appears to have a somewhat different side-effect profile than the other SSRIs, which makes it preferred for some patients. It usually is more sedating and less likely to cause agitation. As with the other SSRIs, headaches, nausea, tiredness, and sexual problems are common side effects.

Drug-Drug Interactions. New-generation antidepressants interact with a number of other medications in complicated and often dangerous ways.

1. *P450 enzyme inhibition.* SSRIs can interfere with the metabolism of common medications. Many different medications are broken apart and made harmless in the liver by a set of enzymes called the P450 system. All SSRIs interfere with these enzymes to varying degrees, which in turn can cause normally prescribed doses of other medications to build up to dangerous levels. To further complicate matters, different SSRIs interfere with different enzymes in the P450 system, which means that different SSRIs interact with different medications. Paroxetine and fluoxetine cause the greatest inhibition of the enzyme that metabolizes tricyclic antidepressants, and they have the largest potential for causing dangerous increases in serum levels when they are taken with medications like desipramine. Fluvoxamine interferes most with the enzyme that metabolizes clozapine. Sertraline, fluoxetine, and nefazodone interfere with the enzyme that metabolizes the common antihistamines terfenadine (Seldane) and astemizole (Hismanal), which can lead to dangerous increases in these normally safe medications.

There are more than 30 specific enzymes in the P450 system, and no one can keep all of the interactions in mind. What is important to remember is that different SSRIs interfere with different parts of this system, and that the serum level of many common medications can increase dramatically when the common medication is given along with an SSRI. Most pharmacists have computer programs that can look for interactions among a list of medications that a patient is taking.

2. *HIV medications.* There are important drug-drug interactions between the SSRI antidepressants and many of the medications used in the treatment of HIV. For example, Norvir and Kaletra both inhibit the enzyme that is used to metabolize fluoxetine, fluvoxamine, venlafaxine, and the tricyclic medications. When used together, the antidepressant should be used at ¼ to ½ of the normal dose. Use of Bupropion (Wellbutrin) can cause even larger, potentially dangerous increases in serum level when taken with these HIV medications. A number of the other HIV medications also have important drug-drug interactions.

3. *Serotonin syndrome.* This is most common and most dangerous when an SSRI is prescribed with an MAOI antidepressant, although it can occur as an interaction with other drugs or even as a side effect of an SSRI alone. Symptoms include confusion, agitation, sweating, increased reflexes, myoclonus (sudden jerking movements), shivering, tremor, coordination problems, fever, and diarrhea. Serotonin syndrome can also occur when SSRIs are taken along with a number of other medications, including dextromethorphan, a very common ingredient in cough medications.

4. *Drug Withdrawal.* People who abruptly stop the SSRIs (and most of the other antidepressants) may have uncomfortable but not dangerous withdrawal symptoms for up to several days or even longer. These withdrawal symptoms can include dizziness, headaches, nausea, vivid dreams, sleep problems, irritability, and paresthesias (feelings of prickling or burning on the skin). These withdrawal symptoms are more common with shorter-activating medication, such as paroxetine and fluvoxamine, and much less common with sertraline and fluoxetine.

Selective Serotonin and Norepinephrine Inhibitor (SSNRI).

1. *Venlafaxine (Effexor)* is a bit different from the SSRIs because, at higher doses, it blocks the reuptake of both serotonin and norepinephrine without blocking other neurotransmitters (at lower doses, it just blocks serotonin and acts like any other SSRI). Some research suggests that venlafaxine may be more effective than the SSRIs. Clinically, venlafaxine may be effective in patients who have not been helped by the pure serotonergic antidepressants, perhaps because it affects two different chemical systems involved in depression.

    Venlafaxine may cause high blood pressure more often than the other SSRIs, especially at doses above 225 mg/day, but it causes less interference with the metabolism of other drugs. Otherwise, the side effects of venlafaxine are very similar to the SSRIs.

    Fluoxetine can interfere with the metabolism of venlafaxine, however, and if a person is switching from one to the other, he or she should start with a very low dose and increase it very gradually over several weeks.

Selective Norepinephrine Reuptake Inhibitor (SNRI).

1. *Reboxetine (Edronax)* (not available in the United States). Reboxetine is already available in Europe, although it is unclear if it will ever be marketed in the United States. It is well tolerated and may work for different people than the already available medications, although some research has suggested that it may be less effective than other standard antidepressants already in use. Reboxetine and other SNRIs may be particularly effective in people who appear to be chronically tired, apathetic, or who have problems with motivation, and these medications may end up being most useful in combination with other SSRI-type antidepressants. Side effects are different than the SSRIs and are related to increased norepinephrine. Common side effects include increased sweating, blurred vision, dry mouth, and insomnia.

Antidepressants that Act Indirectly on Serotonin and Norepinephrine. A number of antidepressants also have action on the serotonin and norepinephrine system through other mechanisms. The exact mechanism of action is not important, except to understand that these other medications may work for people who do not respond to the SSRIs, and that the side effects are different than the SSRIs. The most important difference is that these antidepressants do not commonly have sexual side effects.

1. *Trazodone (Desyrel)* is less effective than other antidepressants as a primary treatment for depression but still has a useful role. Trazodone is very sedating and is often given at night as a mild, safe, nonaddicting sleep aid. In fact, trazodone is sometimes prescribed to help people overcome sleep difficulties caused by activating antidepressants like Prozac. Trazodone is a short-acting medication with a half-life of about 3½ hrs. This means that for most people there is no hangover or lingering effects the next day. A typical dose of trazodone is 50–600 mg/day. Often 50 or 100 mg at bedtime will not interfere with another antidepressant that the person may also be taking.

The most serious problem with trazodone is priapism (very painful, long-lasting erections of the penis), which can require surgery and cause permanent impotence. Any man prescribed trazodone should be warned to stop taking the medication if he experiences any unusual or prolonged erections.

Trazodone has almost no anticholinergic effect, although it does cause dry mouth through a different mechanism. Trazodone is also less likely than the tricyclic antidepressants to potentiate heart block (a block of the electrical impulses between different parts of the heart) in people with preexisting heart disease, although it can increase heart irritability and increase abnormal heartbeats in someone with a preexisting heart disease. Trazodone is much safer in overdoses than the older medications and causes less orthostatic hypotension.

2. *Nefazodone (Serzone)* is similar to trazodone but seems more effective because it has several active metabolites that are better antidepressants than the parent medication. It works through a somewhat different mechanism than any of the other antidepressants. Nefazodone is given in a 300–600 mg/ day dose range. Because some of the metabolites have a short half-life, twice-a-day dosing is indicated. It is generally started at 50–100 mg twice a day and then increased.

Nefazodone has relatively few side effects. Some people report sedation, nausea, dizziness, and anticholinergic side effects, including dry mouth, constipation, and blurred vision. As with the SSRIs, patients can experience headaches and nausea. Nervousness, weight loss, and palpitations all seem less common with nefazodone. *The incidence of sexual side effects is very low—much lower than with many other antidepressants.* Nefazodone also has very little tendency to cause weight gain. It has some significant drug-drug interactions with the antihistamines terfenadine (Seldane) and astemizole (Hismanal) and with cisapride (Propulsid), which is a common medication for gastrointestinal disorders like severe chronic nausea, heartburn, or gastric reflux.

The FDA has recently issued a warning about the very rare but very serious risk of nefazodone causing life-threatening liver failure. It appears that liver failure occurs approximately once in every 250,000 patient-years of people taking nefazodone. While this is a very low rate, it is three to four times the estimated rate for liver failure of people without any known risk. Regular testing of liver function does not appear to be helpful, but early recognition of symptoms and testing if there is concern can be life-saving. Symptoms of liver failure include jaundice, loss of appetite, increasing malaise. Nefazodone should be stopped if liver enzymes (ALT or AST) are more than three times the upper limits of normal. Nefazodone should be used with caution in people with active liver disease.

3. *Mirtazapine (Remeron)* is a newer antidepressant that affects

both serotonin and norepinephrine, to varying degrees depending on the dose. It is often more sedating in lower doses than in higher doses, which means that people may have fewer side effects if it is started at full dose rather than gradually increased the way most medications are. Mirtazapine seems to help the anxiety and the sleep problems common to depression and has minimal sexual side effects. Mirtazapine is typically started at 15 or 30 mg before bed and can be increased to 60 mg or even higher.

Side effects include sedation and increased appetite. Weight gain is much more frequent and can be more significant with mirtazapine than with other antidepressants. Weight gain usually begins early: if it does not start within the first six weeks, it probably will not happen later. On the other hand, *there are virtually no sexual side effects.* Dizziness can be an uncommon problem, especially when the medication is first started. It has relatively mild anticholinergic side effects, including dry mouth and constipation. It seems to have relatively few drug-drug interactions and seems relatively safe in overdoses. According to early research, slightly more than one person in a thousand on mirtazapine stops or decreases production of white blood cells.

Dopamine and Norepinephrine Reuptake Blocker

1. *Bupropion (Wellbutrin)* is the only available antidepressant that acts on dopamine nerve cells. It is reputed to have fewer side effects than the older antidepressants. It has fewer anticholinergic side effects (dry mouth, blurred vision, constipation) than the tricyclic antidepressants. It causes fewer blood pressure problems and has less effect on the electrical activity of the heart. It is also an activating rather than a sedating medication and does not seem to cause the weight gain associated with tricyclics. It is safer than tricyclics if taken in an overdose. Other than dangerous interactions with MAOIs, it has relatively few drug-drug side effects.

Side Effects. The big advantage of bupropion is that it does not cause any sexual side effects. It can sometime reverse the sexual side effects caused by other medications, and it is sometimes given along with an SSRI to both enhance the effectiveness of the first medication and decrease the sexual side effects. It also causes no weight gain in most people.

Bupropion is activating rather than sedating. This means that it does not cause tiredness, but it also does not help with sleep and is not useful for anxiety disorders. It often feels like taking caffeine, and it can be used as a mild stimulant for attention deficit disorder. Common side effects include restlessness and sleep problems. Nausea and tremors are possible but rare.

Bupropion's introduction was delayed because of a high incidence of seizures in several people, all of whom had anorexia. Bupropion's side effects include a higher incidence of seizures, estimated at four times that of most other antidepressants. The seizure incidence is dose-related and increases tenfold when the dose is increased to 450–600 mg/day. Despite this, the risk of seizures is reduced if the person does not have other risks for seizures or is not taking a larger than recommended dose.

Specifics of Use. A normal dose of bupropion is around 300 mg/day, usually divided into three 100-mg doses. To decrease the risk of seizure, no single dose should exceed 150 mg. Bupropion is typically started at 100 mg twice a day and increased no sooner than every three days.

A longer-acting version of bupropion (Wellbutrin SR) is now available. Up to 400 mg of the long-acting bupropion can be given as 200 mg twice a day, rather than taking the medication three times a day as regular bupropion at that dose requires. The incidence of seizures is reported to be less with the long-acting bupropion. The longer-acting bupropion has lower peak levels of medication and therefore affects the dopamine system somewhat less than the standard bupropion. Some people may not respond as well with the long-acting medication, but the increased safety, increased convenience, and decreased risk make the long-acting form the choice of most people.

Bupropion has also been effective in helping people to stop smoking. It seems to stop the craving associated with smoking withdrawal and works best when given along with a nicotine patch and as part of a smoking cessation program. One typically sets a "stop smoking day" 7–10 days after starting bupropion. Patients participating in smoking cessation studies started at 150 mg/day for three days and then increased to 150 mg twice a day.

Tricyclic Antidepressants

Most of the antidepressants used prior to the last few years were "tricyclics" (having a three-ring molecular structure). They include amitriptyline (Elavil), nortriptyline (Pamelor), desipramine (Norpramin), and doxepin (Sinequan).

These older antidepressants are at least as effective (and sometimes more effective) as any of the newer medications for treatment of depression. They are less useful for treatment of OCD and some of the other anxiety disorders. The major problem with these older medications is that they are much more dangerous, especially in overdoses. A month's worth of any of these older medications is lethal if taken all at once. These older medications also make people feel "drugged" and sedated much more than the newer medications.

Side Effects.

1. *Tricyclic antidepressants are all extremely dangerous when taken as an overdose*, and a severely depressed, potentially suicidal client should not be given more than a week's supply of a tricyclic antidepressants without careful consideration. All of the newer antidepressants, such as venlafaxine (Effexor), fluoxetine (Prozac), and sertraline (Zoloft), are much safer if taken as an overdose.

2. *The tricyclic antidepressants potentiate the effect of alcohol,* and a few drinks may make a person taking these medications more intoxicated than he or she would normally get. In addition, alcohol increases the lethality of antidepressants, and a normally nonlethal overdose may become lethal if combined with alcohol.

3. *Anticholinergic side effects are common.* All the traditional, tricyclic antidepressants block the action of acetylcholine and produce the kind of autonomic side effects (side effects related to the involuntary part of the nervous system responsible for basic system regulation) typical of other anticholinergic medications. These include dry mouth, blurred vision, constipation, and, in rare cases, urinary retention, heart palpitations, or tachycardia (speeding pulse) and increased sweating. These medications can, on rare occasions, aggravate certain kinds of glaucoma (increased pressure in the eyeball) and eye pain, which can be helped by special eye drops.

   Anticholinergic medications can also cause confusion and delirium, especially in elderly people who may be taking a number of different medications with anticholinergic side effects.

4. *Cardiovascular side effects include orthostatic hypotension, increased pulse, and EKG changes.* The most serious of these side effects are sudden cardiac arrhythmias (irregularities of the heartbeat) or heart block, when the electrical impulses cannot spread through the heart normally. Sudden death has been reported, but it is extremely rare. Overall, the effects on the heart are very complicated and not all bad. The tricyclic antidepressants (e.g., amitriptyline, desipramine) act on the heart very much like quinidine, a medication used to stabilize certain kinds of heartbeat irregularities. In fact, a person with heart problems who normally requires quinidine can often reduce or eliminate his or her dose if he or she begins taking one of these antidepressants.

5. *Neurological complications are fairly rare.* Grand mal seizures can be caused by all the tricyclic antidepressants. Two newer

antidepressants, bupropion (Wellbutrin) and maprotiline (Ludiomil), seem to have a somewhat higher incidence of seizures than the tricyclics, while all the other newer antidepressants have a much lower seizure frequency. Other side effects of the tricyclics include drowsiness, slurred speech, and hand tremor. Like any other medication with anticholinergic properties, these medications can also cause confusion or even delirium that may be difficult to distinguish from a psychotic episode.

6. *Weight gain is a common problem caused by all of the tricyclic and MAOI antidepressants.* The newer antidepressants, including bupropion (Wellbutrin) and the serotonin-blocking antidepressants (fluoxetine and sertraline), do not normally cause significant weight gain.

7. *Many antidepressants, including the tricyclics, can cause decreased libido and impotence.* They can also block menstrual periods, although this seems less common. Decreasing the dose or switching antidepressants may solve these problems.

8. *All antidepressant medications can trigger a manic episode* in some susceptible people. This may be more likely with the tricyclics than with the newer antidepressants. In addition, some people with schizophrenia reportedly become more disorganized or more paranoid when taking antidepressants. These medications can also cause some people to start "rapid cycling," to have rapid mood swings more than once a month.

9. *Various allergies can also occur,* and any person on any medication who reports a new rash should have it investigated. Also, as with the antipsychotic medications, agranulocytosis (a sudden block in white blood cell production) has been reported. If a person on one of these medications develops a sore throat, sudden chills, or fever, a physician should be alerted and a complete blood count (CBC) should be drawn immediately.

10. *Abrupt withdrawal of these medications sometimes produces nausea, vomiting, abdominal cramps, diarrhea, chills, insom-*

nia, and anxiety lasting three to five days. This withdrawal is not medically dangerous but can be uncomfortable. These medications usually should be withdrawn gradually over several weeks or even longer, especially if the person has been taking the medication for some time.

11. *While these medications usually help sleep, occasionally they produce nightmares.* This can be controlled by lowering the dose, taking the medication earlier in the day, or taking it in divided doses. Agitation and nervousness are uncommon but have been reported.

Specifics of Use. For anyone under 16 or over 40 or anyone who has a history of heart problems, a preliminary EKG is required before starting a tricyclic antidepressant. If there is any possibility of heart disease, a medical clearance should be obtained as well. The usual starting dose for imipramine (Tofranil) and amitriptyline (Elavil) is 50–75 mg/day for two to three days, although in older or physically ill people much lower initial doses can be used. If there are no serious side effects, gradually increase the dose to 150–300 mg/day. It takes from five days to three weeks for these medications to be effective, and a reasonable clinical trial is at least three weeks of medication in doses above 150 mg/day. After the dose is stabilized, most or all of the medication can be given right before bedtime to minimize the sedative and other side effects and to insure a good night's sleep.

It is now possible to determine how much medication is actually present in the body. One person may have ten times the serum level of another person taking the same daily dose of medication. For some medications, such as nortriptyline, there appears to be a "therapeutic window"; that is, serum levels within a certain range (50–150 mg/ml) are more effective than levels below or above this range. For other antidepressants, lower levels seem ineffective while higher levels are, except for their higher side effects, okay. While we now can measure the serum levels of most antidepressants, there still is too little research for us to fully understand what the serum levels mean and how much medication is too much. Other antidepressants like Prozac can interfere with the metabolism of many other medications, including tricyclic antidepressants. This means that if a medication like Prozac is prescribed along with a tricyclic such as desipramine, a normal dose of desipramine can rapidly increase to a dangerous serum level. The same thing can happen if a patient is rapidly switched from Prozac to desipramine.

Monoamine Oxidase Inhibitors (MAOIs)

MAOIs include phenelzine (Nardil) and tranylcypromine (Parnate). They block the action of the enzyme that deactivates neurotransmitters with a single amine group, hence their name mono (one) amine oxidase inhibitors. Some people who have not responded to other medications will respond to MAOIs. MAOIs seem to be particularly useful in people with "atypical depression." These people often have problems with anxiety and agoraphobic symptoms, have weight gain instead of the more common weight loss, and sleep too much instead of too little. Some researchers suggest that people with "hysteroid dysphoria," a vague constellation of symptoms and marked sensitivity to rejection, may respond specifically to MAOIs. Others feel that people with bulimia and agoraphobia may respond better to these medications than to traditional antidepressants.

Side Effects.

1. *The most common serious side effect is a hypertensive crisis* (very rapid, very high, and dangerous elevation of blood pressure). This reaction is caused by an interaction between the MAOI and foods containing tyramine, or between the MAOI and medications that have sympathomimetic effects (effects on the sympathetic nervous system). The MAOIs work by interfering with the enzyme that breaks apart certain neurotransmitters. This same enzyme also breaks apart tyramine, an amino acid that naturally occurs in certain

foods. Since the MAOI keeps this tyramine from being deactivated, it can rapidly accumulate to high levels and cause the increase in blood pressure.

The symptoms of a hypertensive crisis include a severe headache, heart palpitations, nausea and vomiting, unexplained nose bleed, and chest pain. A blood pressure check can quickly determine whether or not there is a problem. Such crises are rare, especially if a person is compliant with the food restrictions, but they can lead to strokes and other catastrophes.

Foods that have high levels of tyramine and must be avoided include:

- Aged cheeses (essentially everything except bland American cheese)
- Smoked or pickled fish
- Chicken liver
- Broad beans (fava beans)
- Chianti and other red wines
- Tap and German beers
- Sauerkraut
- Sausage, salami, and other aged meat
- Dried, salted fish
- Any food that is not fresh

In addition, a large number of additional foods, including chocolate, yogurt, and sour cream, have moderate levels of tyramine and can cause a reaction in some people, especially if eaten in large amounts. A variety of aged foods, such as overripe bananas, can cause problems, as can monosodium glutamate, soy sauce, and meat tenderizer.

2. *MAOIs interact with a large number of other medications*, often in dangerous ways. For example, extremely dangerous interactions occur when Demerol is taken by someone also taking an MAOI. Dextromethorphan, found in many over-the-counter cough medications, is also dangerous. A potentially fatal "serotonin reaction" can occur when MAOIs are given along with SSRIs and other antidepressants that affect

serotonin. Because Prozac has a long half-life, a person should not take an MAOI until he or she has been off Prozac for at least five weeks.

Many nonprescription cold and allergy medications and asthma medications can cause a hypertensive reaction, as can stimulants such as amphetamines and cocaine. People taking MAOIs are strongly advised to check with their doctor or pharmacist about medication interactions before taking any other medication, whether prescribed or over-the-counter. They should also let all treating physicians, dentists, and other health care providers know exactly what medications they are on. Some form of emergency notification, such as a card in their wallet or I.D. bracelet, is also a useful precaution.

3. *MAOIs can also cause orthostatic hypotension.* This can cause temporary dizziness or even fainting, and often the use of the medication must be limited.

4. *MAOIs are activating rather than sedating medications for most people.* This is often an advantage, since they usually do not cause the sedation that is common with other antidepressants, but this activating effect can interfere with sleep. Most people prefer to take these medications early in the day rather than at night, when tricyclics are usually taken. At times it is useful to give low-dose trazodone at night if sleep disturbance is a significant problem. Some people do get sedated from the MAOIs, and feeling lethargic a few hours after taking the medication is not uncommon.

5. *Other side effects are usually less of a problem and less common.* Constipation or diarrhea is sometimes reported, as is dry mouth, transient impotence, skin rash, and blurred vision, despite the fact that MAOIs are not anticholinergic. Serious liver toxicity is rare but has been reported with phenelzine (Nardil).

6. *As with other antidepressants, problems can occur if an MAOI is stopped abruptly.* Withdrawal symptoms include confusion, irritability, agitation, depression, and manic symptoms.

Specifics of Use. A person must be off all other antidepressants for at least ten days before starting a MAOI (people must be off fluoxetine [Prozac] for five weeks). Similarly, if a person switches from one MAOI to another, there must be at least a ten-day medication-free period. The dose of the medication is gradually increased over a week or two, and as with the other antidepressants it usually takes three weeks or longer for the medication to be effective.

DECIDING WHICH ANTIDEPRESSANT TO USE

All of the antidepressants currently available seem equally effective, although a particular medication may be dramatically more effective than another for a particular individual. Unfortunately, there is no way to be certain about which medication will work for which client. Physicians are often inclined to select certain antidepressants because they are familiar with them. It is reasonable to select the medication with the side-effect profile that is least troublesome to the particular client. The main side effects to consider are degree of sedation, degree of anticholinergic activity, cardiovascular side effects (including orthostatic hypotension), and sexual side effects. For example, desipramine is only mildly sedating and has relatively few anticholinergic side effects (dry mouth, blurred vision, etc.). This might be a good medication to choose for people who have had problems with sedation or blurred vision. Fluoxetine (Prozac) might be the medication of choice if no sedation can be tolerated. Fluoxetine usually does not cause much weight gain, but it increases anxiety in some susceptible people. Doxepin (Sinequan), on the other hand, is very sedating, and for people with insomnia this medication's sedative "side effect" might be useful if there is little risk of an overdose. If sexual side effects are of concern, bupropion (Wellbutrin) or nefazodone (Serzone) might be the best choice.

When the first antidepressant does not work and a second medication is being considered, it makes sense to choose a second medication as different as possible from the first, although there are few hard data to support this theory. All types of antidepressants have somewhat different mechanisms of action. Occasionally, a client will respond to one medication and not another even though the medications are of the same type.

Mood-stabilizing medications, such as lithium, are often used to increase the effectiveness of an antidepressant if the antidepressant alone is not fully effective. A number of other augmentation strategies also work well, including combining different antidepressants with different mechanisms of action, using thyroid hormone even when there appears to be normal thyroid function. While there appears to be anecdotal support for these strategies, there is little controlled research demonstrating which of these strategies is most effective for whom.

TABLE 8. Side Effects of Antidepressant Medications

	Sedation	Insomnia	Dry Mouth	Constipation	Orthostatic Hypotension	GI Distress	Weight Gain	Sexual Problems
amitriptyline	+++	+	+++	+	+	+	+++	+
bupropion	0	+	+	+	0	+	0	0
citalopram	+	+	+	0	0	++	++	++
fluoxetine	+	+	+	0	+	++	+	+++
fluvoxamine	+	+	+++	+	0	+++	++	+++
mirtazapine	+++	0	+++	+	0	0	+++	0
nefazodone	++	0	+	+	+	+	0	0
nortriptyline	++	0 to +	++	+	0 to +	0 to +	+	0 to +
paroxetine	+	+	++	+	+	++	++	+++
sertraline	+	+	+	0	+	+++	0 to +	+++
venlavaxine	+	+	+	+	+	+++	0	+++

+mild ++moderate +++severe

5

Mood-Stabilizing Medications

The classic mood stabilizer is lithium. First used in 1949 as an anti-manic treatment, it was the first modern "wonder drug" in psychiatry. In addition to lithium, a number of medications initially developed to control seizures are now commonly used as mood stabilizers. Valproate (Depakote) and carbamazepine (Tegretol) were the first anticonvulsants to also be effective mood stabilizers. Recently, a number of newer anticonvulsants, including gabapentin, topirimine, lamotrigine, and oxcarbazepine, have also been found effective in helping people stabilize their moods.

Mood stabilizers are not "uppers" or "downers" or simple antidepressants. They stabilize both the highs and the lows of some people with mood swings. Mood swings do not always disappear, but they often become less frequent and less severe. In general, mood stabilizers treat classic bipolar disorder, with mood swings occurring less than twice a year, better than they treat rapid cycling disorder or other more atypical mood disorders.

Manic depressive disorder and bipolar disorder are different names for the same disease. While people are manic, they typically are grandiose, are very energetic, need very little sleep, talk very rapidly, often spend money recklessly or engage in other impulsive behavior, are sometimes very irritable, and generally are thinking so fast that they have trouble functioning in normal activities. People who are hypomanic are less out of control, and while they may be thinking and talking rapidly they are generally able to function at work and at home.

LITHIUM

Indications for Use

Lithium is the medication of choice for the helping to control the mood swings in someone who has a manic-depressive or bipolar illness. It decreases the frequency and severity of the manic episodes, but it does not necessarily eliminate them in all people. It is also useful in aborting the acute manic attack and is often used in combination with one of the antipsychotic medications. The antipsychotic slows the person down to a manageable level while the lithium aborts the manic attack itself.

There is also increasing evidence that lithium is useful in schizoaffective disorder and even in some people with schizophrenia who are agitated or aggressive. People who are hyperactive and have pressured speech should be considered as potential lithium candidates, even if they carry a schizophrenic diagnosis. A certain percentage of lithium responders previously have been given a diagnosis of schizophrenia. These people may have carried a schizophrenic diagnosis for many years, and they may have all the first-rank symptoms of schizophrenia. It makes sense to seriously consider a trial of lithium for those with schizophrenia who do not respond well to more traditional therapy and for those who are irritable, angry, or aggressive, all of which are affective symptoms. Whenever a medication is first begun and especially when initiating such trials, it is important to remember that they are just that—trials. The medication should be started and continued for a specified period of time, usually four to six weeks, and target symptoms that were clearly identified before the trial should be followed.

A family history of manic-depressive disorder, depression, or suicide increases the probability that a person is a lithium responder, and it is suggested that a family history of alcoholism might also be a positive sign. A person who reports experiencing depressions and "highs," bouts of excessive spending, or frequent, impulsive marriages should be considered as possibly having manic periods.

Lithium is also helpful in preventing the depressive side of manic-depressive disease and recurrent depression. Recent research has indicated that combining lithium and antidepressants is very effective in treating some people who have never responded to antidepressants alone. Many people with borderline and other personality disorders show marked and at times rapid mood changes, from sad to elated and back again. For some people, lithium or one of the other mood stabilizers will help decrease the number and intensity of these mood fluctuations.

Lithium also has been effective in some people with explosive, uncontrollable anger that does not leave time for the person to consider the consequences of his or her behavior.

Side Effects

1. *Effects on the kidney.* Lithium is excreted by the kidneys and preexisting kidney disease (determined by BUN and serum creatinine tests) can allow a dangerous buildup of the medication in a short time. Increased fluid intake and urination are common in most people on lithium because of its direct effect on the kidneys, causing a syndrome called nephrogenic diabetes insipides. In some rare cases, this increased urination may be severe enough to cause serious dehydration. For almost all individuals, these kidney effects can be inconvenient, but they rarely cause actual kidney damage and usually correct themselves when the medication is discontinued. Very few people on long-term lithium therapy incur permanent, irreversible, and potentially life-threatening kidney damage. No clear information about the frequency of such damage is available, except that it seems to be rare and can be prevented by discontinuing lithium before the kidney

damage gets too severe. All people on lithium should have their serum creatinine measured every 6–12 months to detect early kidney damage.

2. *Thyroid effects.* Lithium is known to interfere with thyroid function and it may be useful to get a yearly TSH (thyroid-stimulating hormone) to test for this. Hypothyroidism (underactive thyroid) often develops very slowly and is easy to miss. It is very important for both clinicians and people taking lithium to be aware of early signs of thyroid dysfunction and obtain a TSH if there is any concern. Signs of decreased thyroid function include weight gain, fatigue, intolerance to cold, constipation, hoarse voice, and rough, dry skin. It is not necessary to stop the lithium, since providing extra thyroid hormone in a daily pill can treat decreased thyroid function easily.

3. *Common, uncomfortable side effects.* The most common side effect of lithium is a fine tremor of hands that usually begins during the first few days of treatment. Nausea, vomiting, mild abdominal pain, fatigue, and thirst are also common initially but usually disappear in a few weeks. These side effects may be decreased by giving the medication in smaller divided doses or giving it along with food so that absorption is slowed. Some weight gain is common, although it is not as frequent or as much as with Depakote or some other medications. A metallic taste in the mouth and frequent urination are other reported symptoms. Lithium can affect the heart and causes minor changes in the EKGs of many people. This is rarely a serious problem. Finally, lithium can cause some people to feel as though their thinking is a bit "fuzzy" or slowed down. At times people report that they feel less creative or a bit numb in how they react emotionally.

4. *Toxic side effects.* Toxic side effects of lithium, which initially look like an exaggeration of the common, nontoxic side effects, include thirst, decreased appetite, vomiting, and diarrhea. However, these can progress to confusion, coarse tremor,

muscle twitching, and slurred speech. In extreme cases, the person appears drunk and has muscle twitches, nystagmus (small jerks of the eye), hyperreflexia (increased reflexes), seizures, stupor, and eventually coma. The neurological symptoms in such cases may be present in only one side of the body or may be more severe on one side than they are on the other. If a person taking lithium develops diarrhea or nausea, lithium intoxication should be considered and serum lithium levels obtained.

Specifics of Use

Before starting lithium, a serum BUN (blood urea nitrogen) and serum creatinine should be obtained to determine that the person's kidneys are working properly. Lithium is excreted by the kidneys, and if they are not working properly the lithium can rapidly build up to toxic levels. An EKG is suggested by some experts but is probably unnecessary, unless there is concern about heart disease. Some experts suggest a creatinine clearance test as well, but this requires collecting all of a person's urine over 24 hours, which is quite cumbersome, expensive, and usually impossible outside of a hospital. Following serum creatinine over the course of lithium therapy is a reasonably safe way to detect early kidney damage. A yearly urinalysis may give some information about the kidneys' ability to concentrate urine, but it is not part of most protocols. Though there is concern about lithium and kidney damage, such damage seems rare.

Lithium can decrease the production of thyroid hormone. This is easily treatable, but people should be aware of the symptoms of decreased thyroid activity (hypothyroidism). A lab test for thyroid function taken every year or so is often recommended.

Start by giving 600–900 mg/day of lithium carbonate in divided doses. Lithium carbonate usually comes in 300-mg capsules, so a typical dose is three to four capsules a day. Lithium was once given two or three times a day because of concern of toxicity and side effects. Recently, it has become apparent that most people do well taking the entire dose at one time, usually at mealtime to decrease gastrointestinal side effects.

Follow with serum lithium levels and adjust the dose so that the lithium level in the blood is 0.6–1.2 meq/l (millequivalents per liter, a measure of concentration). The textbooks used to suggest that lithium levels be 0.8–1.2 meq/l. Recent research has suggested that people have fewer relapses if their lithium is kept between 0.8 and 1.0 meq/l than if their level is allowed to drop to the 0.4–0.6 meq/l range. Unfortunately, they also have poorer compliance and more side effects at the higher levels. While there is some increased risk of relapse at the lower dose, for some people the decrease in side effects may make this risk worthwhile. Most people require 600–1,800 mg/day to maintain their serum lithium level within this therapeutic range. Older people and people with brain damage generally require less lithium and, in fact, may become toxic on normal doses. Usually, as a person ends a manic episode, less medication is needed to maintain the same serum medication level. People who have had a stable lithium level while manic may become toxic if they continue to take the same amount of lithium after they calm down. Conversely, people going into a manic episode will frequently need to increase their daily lithium dose to maintain a therapeutic serum lithium level.

After a person seems stable on a given dose of lithium, blood levels should be measured at least every six months. Blood levels change during the day, peaking several hours after the person takes a dose and dropping slowly until the next dose. It is important, therefore, to standardize when the blood sample is drawn. A serum level of 0.6 meq/l 12 hours after a dose means something different from the same level 24 hours after a dose. Standard serum levels should always be taken 12 hours after a normal dose of medication is taken. A person receiving divided doses of lithium should have his or her lithium level checked before taking his or her morning dose, which should be about 12 hours after the evening dose was taken.

Some of the side effects from lithium can be treated. Mild diarrhea can be treated by over-the-counter medications, such as Kaopectate. A fine intention tremor can be treated with low-dose propranolol, which is relatively safe, easy to use, and effective. Still, using one medication to treat the side effects of another only makes sense when the tremor is causing some problem or discomfort. If increased urination becomes a serious problem for a person taking lithium, because it is either dehydrating or so frequent that it is interfering with the person's life, hydrochlorothiazide may be prescribed. This is a diuretic that normally causes people to urinate more but works paradoxically on people suffering from increased urination because of lithium. There is some concern that hydrochlorothiazide may increase the risk of kidney damage from lithium, and it is only used when the increased urinary frequency is severe. Hydrochlorothiazide increases most people's serum lithium levels, potentially to toxic levels. To prevent lithium toxicity, the dose of lithium is usually decreased at the same time that hydrochlorothiazide is started, and serum lithium levels are monitored carefully. Hydrochlorothiazide also causes potassium loss, which needs to be monitored.

People who are alcoholic and are taking lithium present a special problem because they may become dehydrated during drinking binges, thereby secondarily increasing their serum lithium levels enough to become toxic. The resulting acute organic brain syndrome might be from lithium as well as alcohol. This seems rare because most people generally stop taking their medications while drinking. However, lithium toxicity should be considered for anyone who is drunk and/or dehydrated while on lithium.

Drug-Drug Interactions

Lithium interacts with a number of commonly prescribed medications. The most common problem is a rise in the serum lithium level, at times to toxic levels, when a person initially stable on lithium begins taking an additional medication. This occurs with hydrochlorothiazide, a very common medication used for water retention and high blood pressure, and with a number of pain medications, including most of the nonsteroidal, anti-inflammatory medications like indomethacin (Indocin), phenylbutazone (Butazolidin), and possibly ibuprofen (Motrin). Aspirin and acetaminophen (Tylenol) are safe.

Use During Pregnancy

There is evidence that lithium increases the risk of serious birth defects, especially if taken during the first three months of pregnancy. This risk is high enough that women who become pregnant or who are planning to become pregnant should stop taking lithium if possible.

Overdoses of Lithium

Lithium is toxic when taken as an overdose. Frequently, a person overdosing on lithium will vomit it up. If the lithium is not vomited up, a high lithium level (above 2.5 meq/l) can cause damage to the nervous system, including the brain and kidneys. Lithium overdoses must be taken very seriously. Prompt treatment can almost always avoid damage, but in some cases treatment includes kidney dialysis to rapidly remove lithium from the person's blood.

Laboratory Monitoring

A screen for pregnancy should be done before starting the medication, either by taking a careful history or by taking a urine test. Most textbooks suggest that a screen for kidney function be done before starting lithium. I feel that when starting lithium in someone who is medically healthy without a history of high blood pressure or kidney disease, it is safe to decrease the number of blood draws by waiting to obtain an initial screen for kidney function (BUN and serum creatinine) until the first lithium level. A lithium level should be obtained approximately five to seven days after starting lithium, and five to seven days after each dose change. For stable patients, a lithium level should be obtained at least every six months and a creatinine level every year. All lithium levels should be drawn approximately 12 hours after the last dose of lithium.

People taking lithium over time may have a decrease in thyroid function. The standard protocol is to test for this before starting lithium and then every year or so. However, if I am trying to minimize tests I simply watch for symptoms of thyroid problems, such as weight gain, depression, a sense of sluggishness, problems tolerating cold, dry skin, and a persistently hoarse voice. If I notice any of these symptoms, I order a TSH (thyroid-stimulating hormone) to assess thyroid at that time.

DIVALPROEX SODIUM (DEPAKOTE) AND VALPROIC ACID (DEPAKENE)

Depakote is divalproex sodium, which is a compound of valproate and valproic acid. Depakene is just valproic acid. The terms valproate, valproic acid, and divalproex sodium are used interchangeably and all are transformed to the exact same chemical in the body, although formally they are slightly different chemicals. When someone refers to a pill of valproate or valproic acid, he or she is simply using shorthand for the term divalproex sodium.

Indications for Use

Divalproex sodium was originally developed as an anticonvulsant, but it is now in widespread use as a mood stabilizer. Both divalproex sodium and lithium carbonate are considered first medications of choice for treatment of manic-depressive illness. Lithium carbonate has been used longer, we have more information about its effectiveness, and it is much cheaper than divalproex sodium. Divalproex sodium can be started at a full dose essentially from the beginning and seems to work more rapidly. Both medications have their own side effects, but for many people the side effects of divalproex sodium are easier to live with than those of lithium.

Divalproex sodium becomes the medication of choice (over lithium) when the symptoms or illness course do not fit into a classic manic-depressive pattern. Divalproex sodium is the medication of choice for people who are rapid cycling (having four or more episodes of mania or depression a year), have extreme mood instability, have a seizure disorder or a history of seizures, or have any history of brain damage. Divalproex sodium is also used to increase the effectiveness of antidepressants and to treat rage reactions (uncontrollable anger).

Side Effects

In general, valproate is well tolerated and allows many people a greater sense of well-being and less restriction of creativity than is sometimes reported with lithium.

Common, Annoying, but Not Medically Dangerous, Side Effects. Weight gain is the biggest common problem with Depakote. This appears to be dose-related. Weight gain occurs in about half of the people using Depakote. There is now a long-acting form of Depakote that, according to the manufacturer, may cause less weight gain, but so far there is little data to support this suggestion.

Nausea, vomiting, and indigestion are common problems when Depakote is first started but usually wear off after a week or two. Depakote (a compound of valproic acid and sodium valproate) is packaged in a coated, time-release pill that seems to cause less gastrointestinal upset than Depakene (valproic acid alone). Sedation has been reported, although this is less common than with carbamazepine. Tremor is listed as a side effect but also seems rare. Hair loss is rare but can be a serious problem for some people. However, hair growth usually resumes even if the medication is continued and may be helped with selenium and zinc mineral supplements.

Medically Dangerous Side Effects. While valproic acid has been associated with serious liver toxicity in children, it is extremely rare in adults. If liver problems are going to occur, it will almost always be in the first six months of use. It is generally safe for people with hepatitis C or other liver problems to use Depakote, but liver function tests should be followed more frequently, depending on the seriousness of the liver problem.

There have been a few reported cases of inflammation of the pancreas connected with Depakote use. This is extremely painful and can, in rare cases, be fatal. The primary symptom of pancreatitis is abdominal pain. Anyone taking Depkote who experiences severe abdominal pain should be evaluated by a physician.

The data is not clear, but Depakote may cause polycystic ovary disease in women of child-bearing age. This can cause endocrine problems, including excess hair growth and decreased fertility.

Specifics for Use

While some people start Depakote slowly and increase gradually over several weeks, it is safe to start it more rapidly. I often start Depakote by prescribing 500-mg tablets twice a day and then obtain a valproate blood level five days later. A normal dose is 1,000–2,000 mg/day, but this is usually adjusted based on blood levels. Occasionally, a much higher dose is required to achieve a therapeutic blood level. It is also safe and well tolerated to begin Depakote at a full dose, usually figured at 15–20 mg/kg. For example, a person who weighs 220 pounds (100 kg) can be safely started on 1,500–2,000 mg/day in divided doses. There is often less nausea if Depakote is started twice a day, but most people can take it once a day without problems after the first week or so.

The effective serum concentrations needed to prevent seizures is 65–125 µg/l. There is much less research on the serum level needed for valproic acid to be an effective mood stabilizer, but it seems more effective when used at the upper end of this range, usually 80–125 µg/l.

It is suggested that liver function tests be obtained every 6–12 months, and serum levels every six months—given the very low frequency of liver problems in adults, however, it is unclear if this is necessary after the first six months.

There is now an extended-release form of Depakote called Depakote ER. Some clinicians have suggested that this form of the medication may have fewer side effects and may even cause less weight gain. This may turn out to be true, but so far there is little data to support this idea.

Drug-Drug Interactions

Depakote can inhibit the metabolism of other commonly used medications. This means that there can be higher serum levels than one would expect. For example, carbamazepine levels, and in particular some of the more bothersome metabolites (break down products), can increase when used along with Depakote, increasing side effects. Depakote can increase the serum levels of tricyclic antidepressants. Depakote also significantly increases the serum levels of lamotrigine (lamictal). The dose of the lamotrigine is typically halved when given along with Depakote.

Use during Pregnancy

Valproate is associated with birth defects, primarily neural tube defects, when taken in the first trimester of a pregnancy. Women starting valproate should be given a pregnancy test or carefully asked about the possibility of pregnancy.

Laboratory Monitoring

A screen for pregnancy should be done before starting the medication, either by taking a careful history or by taking a urine test. I get a WBC (white blood count) with differential and liver tests at the time of the first blood level, usually five to seven days after starting the medication. I will get another WBC and liver function test in a month or two if I need another serum level, but if I have no clinical concern I may go up to six months for the next WBC and liver function tests, with yearly monitoring after that.

CARBAMAZEPINE (TEGRETOL)

Indications for Use

Carbamazepine (Tegretol) is useful for people with a manic-depressive illness who do not respond well to lithium or valproic acid or who cannot tolerate the side effects of these other medications. Carbamazepine can be used along with both lithium and valproic acid. It seems particularly useful for people with atypical illness or rapid cycling manic-depressive disorder, with more than two episodes a year. It has also been used successfully in certain people with very resistant depressions, usually in combination with other medications.

Carbamazepine is also being used in a variety of other conditions where lithium and valproic acid have been ineffective. Some people with schizophrenia whose ongoing affective lability makes stabilization difficult respond well to either lithium or carbamazepine in combination with an antipsychotic medication. People with aggressive or violent outbursts also seem to respond to carbamazepine or one of the other mood-stabilizing medications. It was once thought that some kind of hidden seizure disorder caused these outbursts, but carbamazepine seems to be effective in people who have no evidence of any kind of seizures.

Side Effects

Common, Annoying, but Not Medically Dangerous, Side Effects. Generally carbamazepine produces less weight gain, hair loss, and tremor than valproic acid, and less tremor, urination, and thirst than lithium. The drawbacks of carbamazepine include increased sedation, a slightly higher incidence of serious side effects, and the potential to be fatal in overdose. Some people also feel confused or drugged by the medication. These are all dose-related side effects and can be minimized by decreasing the dose.

Sedation is common, as is a drunk-like sense of clumsiness. These side effects are dose-related and tend to get better within a few days if the person keeps taking the medication.

Nausea is common when the medication is first started, but tends to get better or disappear within a week or so.

Medically Dangerous Side Effects. Carbamazepine can interfere with the production of white blood cells and can cause leukopenia. This usually develops over time, and the white count rarely drops to a dangerous level. On very rare occasions (four cases per million patients), the body entirely stops making white blood cells (agranulocytosis). This is reversible if diagnosed in time but fatal if allowed to continue. Regular white blood counts are not very useful in preventing the abrupt development of agranulocytosis, but they will indicate any gradual decrease in white cell counts. *Any person taking carbamazepine who gets an infection, fever, sore throat, or mouth sores should immediately get a CBC (complete blood count).*

Liver problems are a rare but potentially dangerous side effect. People taking carbamazepine should be alert to any symptoms of hepatitis, including abdominal tenderness under the right ribs or having the skin or the whites of the eyes turn yellow. Rashes are relatively common and can, on rare occasions, lead to serious problems. Generally the medication does not need to be stopped if a mild rash develops, as long as there is no associated fever, bleeding, or peeling blisters (exfoliative rash).

Temporary increases in liver enzymes are fairly common. Generally liver function tests should be monitored, but the medication does not need to be stopped unless they are twice the normal values.

Specifics of Use

Carbamazepine is usually started at 100–200 mg twice a day, and the dose is increased until the serum level is 5–12 μg/l. Some people who appear confused or sedated, despite having a normal serum level, have a buildup of an active metabolite of carbamazepine called 10,11 epoxide. This, too, can be measured if there is any clinical concern. It takes approximately five days for a dose change to show up fully in a serum level. Carbamazepine induces liver enzymes. That is, the liver gets used to breaking it down, which makes the level tend to drop over the first six weeks or so, even if the same dose is taken. (Alcohol does the same thing, which is one of the reasons seasoned drinkers can drink more without getting as drunk.)

Drug-Drug Interactions. Carbamazepine "induces" many liver enzymes. That is, over a few weeks, it gets the liver to increase the ability to deactivate both carbamazepine and other medications. This can lower the blood level of these other medications. *As a result, carbamazepine can interfere with the effectiveness of many oral contraceptives.* Serum levels of many antipsychotics such as haloperidol are decreased when carbamazepine is started. It lowers lamotrigine levels, and a lamotrigine dose is generally doubled when given along with carbamazepine. Erythromycin, cimetidine, and SSRI antidepressants can all increase the serum level of carbamazepine. Carbamazepine should not be used in combination with clozapine. There is a concern that the combination may increase the risk of agranulocytosis.

Use During Pregnancy. Carbamazepine is associated with birth defects, especially during the first trimester. Birth defects caused by carbamazepine include neural tube defects, defects in the face and skull, underdevelopment of fingernails, and developmental delay. Women starting carbamazepine should be given a pregnancy test or carefully asked about the possibility of being pregnant.

Laboratory Monitoring. Carbamazepine can interfere with white blood cell production. It is important to instruct patients about the warning signs of a dangerous decrease in white blood cell production. Any patient on carbamazepine, especially during the first six months, who has a fever, sore throat, or symptoms of a flu should immediately have a white blood count obtained.

Most textbooks suggest assessing white blood cell production before starting any medication. Certainly, a baseline pre-medication WBC (white blood count) can be useful. If I am trying to minimize blood tests and the person is healthy, I feel it is reasonably safe to get both the first WBC with differential and initial screen for liver problems (SGOT, SGPT, LDH) at the time the first blood level is taken, approximately five days after starting the medication. I get a repeat WBC every time I get a blood level, which usually is several times in the first month of treatment. I then try to get a repeat WBC with differential and liver function test at 3 months, at 6 months, and at least every 12 months thereafter. Carbamazepine auto-induces enzymes, which means that the serum level tends to drop during the first couple months and needs to be monitored more frequently at the beginning. All carbamazepine levels should be drawn approximately 12 hours after the last dose of carbamazepine.

A screen for pregnancy should be done before starting the medication, either by taking a careful history or by taking a urine test.

NEWER MOOD STABILIZERS

There is relatively little research supporting the use of the newer mood stabilizers, but all of them are increasingly being used as back-up medications when the first-line medications either do not work or have intolerable side effects. There is a general belief that these medications are more effective in people with rapid cycling or atypical mood disorders, and they may be less useful in people with classical bipolar disorder. As we learn more, the uses of these newer medications will probably change. We may find out that some are really effective and safe, and we may find that some in this list are less useful and become used less.

Gabapentin (Neurotin)

Gabapentin is a new-generation anticonvulsant that seems to be helpful in a number of psychiatric conditions including anxiety disorders and social phobia. It is widely used by neurologists for neurogenic pain and for treatment of headaches. In addition, it seems to have mood-stabilizing properties. There is little research support for gabapentin as a mood stabilizer, and trials using it in classic manic-depressive illness have been negative. At the same time, it seems useful in helping people with rapid cycling or mood lability. It seems generally well tolerated and safe (even in overdose).

Side Effects. Gabapentin is very safe and well tolerated. It can cause sedation, tiredness, or dizziness in some people, but these effects are relatively rare. In high doses it can cause some weight gain, but this is less common and less severe than with many other mood stabilizers. It has few drug-drug interactions.

Specifics of Use. Gabapentin is used over a wide dose range, from 100 mg twice a day to 1,200 mg four times a day. Blood tests do not help find the best dose. Generally one starts at 300 mg once or twice a day and then increases the dose by 300 mg every few days until it seems to work. It is a very safe medication and can be started at a much higher dose if necessary. It should be given multiple times a day because it has a short half-life.

Lamotrigine (Lamictal)

Lamotrigine seems to be effective for people with rapid-cycling bipolar disorder, hard-to-treat mixed states, and rapid cycling caused by antidepressants. It seems particularly useful in treating the depression that is a common component of atypical mood disorders. It is less effective as an antimanic medication, but it seems much more effective than the others for the depressive end of a mood swing. It can be safely combined with other mood stabilizers, although dose adjustments must be made to compensate for drug-drug interactions when used with either carbamazepine or valproate.

Side Effects. Lamotrigine is usually very well tolerated. Dizziness or double vision are occasionally reported but are rare. Headaches are sometimes reported but seem to go away over a few days if the medication is continued. The biggest problem is with a rash that develops in up to 10% of people taking lamotrigine. *If a rash develops, the lamotrigine should be stopped immediately.* Usually the rash then goes away without problems. In rare cases, especially if the medication is continued, this rash can lead to a potentially fatal condition called Stevens Johnson syndrome.

Specifics of Use. It is very important to start lamotrigine at a very low dose and increase very slowly. The biggest risk is a dangerous rash. This rash seems related to how fast the medication is started. Unfortunately, it takes a long time for someone to get on an effective dose of lamotrigine.

Generally start with 25 mg/day (12.5 mg for people on valproic acid) and increase by 25 mg every week or two. Increasing the dose more rapidly seems to increase the risk of developing a rash. A typical dose is 100–200 mg/day for people on lamotrigine alone. Because of enzyme induction, a higher dose may be required if lamotrigine is taken along with carbamazepine. Because of enzyme inhibition, a lower dose is usually needed if taken with valproic acid.

Oxcarbazepine (Trileptil)

Oxcarbazepine is one of the metabolites, or break-down products, of carbamazepine. When carbamazepine is broken apart in the body it breaks into pieces that continue to be active. One of these pieces is responsible for much of the sedation, confusion, and effect on the liver and on white blood cells

caused by carbamazepine. Another active metabolite of carbamazepine is oxcarbazepine. The break-down products from
oxcarbazepine are all inactive. The hope is that oxcarbazepine
has all of the effectiveness of the original carbamazepine, but
with fewer side effects. It is clear that oxcarbazepine has fewer
side effects than carbamazepine, but there is ongoing debate
about whether it is as effective. While oxcarbazepine is becoming used more widely as a mood stabilizer, at this moment
there is little research clearly showing that it is effective.

Side Effects. Oxcarbazepine has many fewer side effects than
   carbamazepine. It seems to cause much less sedation and
   confusion than does carbamazepine. It can induce liver enzymes and lower the blood levels of other medications, including birth control pills, but this effect is much less than
   that of carbamazepine. It probably can cause the same problems with the liver and with decreasing production of white
   blood cells as does carbamazepine, but these seem less severe and less frequent.

Specifics of Use. There is little information about the best dose
   of oxcarbazepine. Typically one starts with 300-mg tablets
   twice a day and then raises the dose as needed until the
   person's mood is more stable or side effects become a problem. The current maximum dose is 2,400 mg/day. Blood levels do not seem very helpful.

Tiagabine (Gabitril)

Tiagabine is a new anticonvulsant that has been proposed as
a mood stabilizer. There is one paper with three case examples,
and there has been some anecdotal support from other individual cases. There is no controlled research, but tiagabine might
be worth trying in an informed person who has already tried
all of the more conventional approaches to dealing with mood
instability. It appears relatively safe and well tolerated. It has
only been used as a mood stabilizer in combination with other

medications, so it is a bit difficult to interpret side effects. The most common reported side effects are dizziness, tiredness, and confusion. Very occasionally, people taking tiagabine for seizures report an increase in depression. All reports of side effects appear rare.

Based on very little experience, it seems that tiagabine as a mood stabilizer requires a lower dose than when used to control seizures. Most case reports start the medication at 4 mg/day, and increase if necessary to 8–12 mg/day. This is in contrast to the dose range of 16–56 mg/day typically used to control seizures. A number of other anticonvulsants have been proposed as mood stabilizers, and as more research is done, more might be added to the list.

Topirimate (Topamax)

Topirimate is one of the very few medications that cause weight loss. It can reverse some of the weight gain caused by other medications, including the weight gain caused by olanzapine and clozapine. Unfortunately, the weight loss is often modest, and may not continue over a period of years. It is also used as a mood stabilizer, but the data is mixed. Some studies and some clinical reports are very positive, while others are less so.

Side Effects. I have heard several people taking Topirimate call it "the stupid pill." It can cause thinking difficulties, specifically problems finding the right word when people are trying to talk and problems with memory. It can also cause kidney stones.

Recently, several cases of glaucoma have been reported in people taking topirimate. While this is rare, it can cause blindness if not treated rapidly. *People taking topirimate should call a physician immediately if eye pain develops or they experience change in vision.* It appears that glaucoma is more of a risk in the first month or two after starting the medication, and the risk decreases thereafter.

Specifics of Use. Topirimate is usually started at 25 mg a day. Some people respond to this low dose for both mood stability and weight loss, while others may need up to 200 mg/day or even more. The side effects are directly related to dose amount and how rapidly the dose is increased.

TABLE 9. *Overview of Common Mood Stabilizers*

	Usual Dose (mg/day)	Serum Level (μg/l)	Side Effects
carbamazepine	400–1,600	4–12	Drowsiness, confusion, dizziness, decrease in white blood cell production, liver problems
gabapentin	900–2,400	n/a	Fatigue, dizziness
lamotrigine	200–400	n/a	Skin rash, nausea
lithium	600–1,800	0.6–1.2	Tremor, diarrhea, weight gain, kidney problems, cognitive difficulty, thyroid problems
topirimate	200–400	n/a	Problems finding words, decreased concentration, kidney stones, glaucoma
valproic acid	750–3,500	50–120	Nausea, weight gain, sedation, tremor, hair loss, liver and pancreas problems

6

Antianxiety and
Sleeping Medications

Almost all of the central nervous system depressants, including alcohol and barbiturates, have antianxiety properties and can be used as tranquilizers. Similarly, these medications all have sedative properties and can be used to aid sleep. Antianxiety medications are sometimes referred to as "minor tranquilizers" to distinguish them from the antipsychotic medications that are sometimes called "major tranquilizers." These names are very misleading. "Minor tranquilizers" are extremely effective and not at all "minor." "Major tranquilizers" are sedating, and therefore have some tranquilizing properties, but are more accurately labeled antipsychotic medications. Antianxiety medications are also referred to as anxiolytic. Sleeping pills are referred to as hypnotics.

The most useful tranquilizers are generally those that have the largest antianxiety effects with the least sedation. The most useful sleeping pills are those that do not cause sedation the next day. At times it is useful to prescribe a medication that will help someone sleep, but will also have antianxiety effects the next day. In this situation, a longer-acting benzodiazepine may be most effective.

BENZODIAZEPINES

Benzodiazepines have largely supplanted older medications like barbiturates. Benzodiazepines include diazepam (Valium), chlordiazepoxide (Librium), clonazepam (Klonopin), alprazolam (Xanax), flurazepam (Dalmane), and many others. These medications are much safer and less addicting than the older medications that they have largely replaced.

The benzodiazepines, barbiturates, and many of the other medications used as sleeping pills or antianxiety medications can be addicting and are subject to abuse. To put this into perspective, all of the antianxiety medications now in widespread use are much less addicting (and much less dangerous) than alcohol.

The benzodiazepines are all at least partially cross-tolerant with each other and with alcohol (an addicted individual can replace one medication with another in that class), and withdrawal from these medications is much more medically dangerous than heroin withdrawal. Abruptly stopping the use of medications in someone who is addicted to alcohol, barbiturates, or diazepam (Valium) can result in life-threatening convulsions. If addiction to any of these medications is a possibility, medication for a gradual detoxification should be prescribed, and hospital admission may be necessary to control drug use.

Indications for Use

The benzodiazepines are most commonly used as antianxiety medications. They are relatively safe medications that are rarely lethal in an overdose, *except when combined with alcohol.* An overdose of a benzodiazepine in someone who is drunk can be extremely dangerous. The benzodiazepines all have anticonvulsant properties—clonazepam (Klonopin) is regularly used as an anticonvulsant, and diazepam (Valium) can be used intravenously to stop a seizure. In those very rare instances when a person must be sedated before you know what is going on, a benzodiazepine, such as diazepam or lorazepam, is a good medication to use, as it is usually safer than antipsychotic medications like Thorazine and Haldol. Street drugs are commonly cut with scopolamine or a similar anticholinergic drug that is made worse by Thorazine, and the street drug PCP, or "angel dust," can have serious lethal interactions with Thorazine.

Diazepam is absorbed faster and more completely by mouth than by intramuscular injection, so it should be given by pill. If a very fast response is required in an emergency situation, 2–4 mg of lorazepam (Ativan) can be given by injection. As with all medications, the benzodiazepines should not be used without a reason and should not be continued without a reason for continuation.

As an antianxiety medication, diazepam (Valium) is commonly prescribed in 5- or 10-mg tablets up to 40 mg/day. Chlordiazepoxide (Librium) is usually prescribed in doses of 10–25 mg up to 100 mg/day. When alprazolam (Xanax) is used as an antianxiety medication, a typical dose range would be 1–4 mg/day given in divided doses. When alprazolam is used as an antipanic medication, it is often necessary to use a significantly higher dose. In most cases, when these medications are used as antianxiety medications, their use should be restricted to short-term (i.e., one to two weeks) for crises or periods of extreme stress. Chronic use has its place, but only rarely. It is clear that many people with a long history of very high chronic anxiety can feel and function much better on a small, ongoing dose of a benzodiazepine. Long-term use is typically not indicated in those who have a history of addiction, who already have a problem with alcohol use, or who increase their dose of the benzodiazepine.

As a detoxification agent in people addicted to other depressant medications, larger doses of Valium or Librium will be needed; the dosage should then change as the person's clinical condition changes. In alcohol withdrawal, using 50 mg of Librium every two hours is not uncommon. Do not add insult to injury by giving diazepam to someone who is still intoxicated with alcohol or barbiturates. At times, those who are accustomed to a high blood alcohol level can go into withdrawal while still having alcohol in their blood, as long as the blood alcohol level is significantly less than that to which they have become tolerant. In these cases, a benzodiazepine may be indicated to treat the withdrawal.

An acutely out-of-control person who might be using street drugs and for whom a good history and diagnosis are not available may have to be sedated when restraints are not enough. In these cases, lorazepam 1–2 mg or diazepam 10–20 mg by mouth may be safer than an antipsychotic. A person with schizophrenia or mania who is both acutely psychotic and out of control can often be sedated with a combination of an antipsychotic medication and a benzodiazepine. This combination helps reestablish control with a lower dose of antipsychotic medication than would otherwise be necessary, often with fewer side effects.

Side Effects

1. *All of the benzodiazepines are clearly addictive.* The short-acting benzodiazepines, e.g., alprazolam (Xanax), are more addicting than the longer-acting medications in the same class. Medications with a "kick" caused by their rapid onset of action, such as Valium, seem somewhat more subject to abuse than medications with a more gradual onset such as Librium. Anyone who has been taking these medications for more than a few days should have his or her meds decreased slowly rather than abruptly discontinued. Serious, at times life-threatening, seizures from abrupt withdrawal have been reported with all of the benzodiazepines, but these are more likely with short-acting than long-acting medications. A gradual withdrawal is safer and will also help minimize the inevitable discomfort that accompanies withdrawal.

2. *All of the benzodiazepines may cause drowsiness* (which usually improves after a few days of use). People should be warned about using machinery or driving cars, especially when getting used to these medications. They also cause a type of intoxication similar to alcohol, with impaired judgment, decreased coordination, light-headedness, etc. Recent research has suggested that even people well adjusted to small doses of these medications have a measurable impairment in their driving ability. With short-acting medications, these effects

wear off quickly; they remain much longer with the longer-acting medications.

3. *Benzodiazepines can sometimes unleash otherwise inhibited violent behavior.* Again, this "disinhibition" is similar to but much less severe than that with alcohol intoxication.

4. *All of these medications can interfere with memory.* This seems to be a particular problem with triazolam (Halcion) and the other short-acting medications, and with older people who might already have some memory impairment.

Use During Pregnancy

It has been suggested that these medications might increase birth defects. Although recent reviews have found no evidence of increased birth defect with these medications, as a precaution they should be avoided by pregnant women, especially during the first three months of pregnancy.

Differences Among Benzodiazepines

In general, the major differences among benzodiazepines are the speed of onset of action and how long the medication's half-life is—that is, the time it takes for the body to eliminate 50% of the medication. These duration effects vary depending on whether the medication is used occasionally or daily. For the occasional user, Valium's duration is limited by redistribution. Valium rapidly leaves active sites on nerve cells and is absorbed by fat cells. After chronic use, these fat cells become saturated, and duration is limited by the speed with which the medication is broken down by the liver, a much longer process. In the occasional user, Valium is a short-acting medication, but for the chronic user it is a very long-acting medication. Oxazepam (Serax) has a shorter duration of action (half-life) than most of the others. Dalmane has a rapid onset and a long half-life, so, although it is sold as a sleeping pill, it has significant anxiolytic (tranquilizing) action for the next day or two. Both Valium and Librium have moderately long half-lives. The effective half-lives of many medications such as Valium are extended by the presence of active metabolites. That is, the medication is broken down into other chemicals that continue to have sedative and anxiolytic effects.

A benzodiazepine that acts rapidly will be felt by the person as "doing something," while a slower-onset medication is often perceived to be less effective because one does not feel a "kick." On the other hand, rapid-onset sedative hypnotics tend to be more addicting than similar medications with a slower onset of action. When a long-acting medication like Dalmane is given to help with sleep, it can cause a significant hangover the next day, and when given several nights in a row, it can build up in the person and cause tiredness or confusion. A hangover can be avoided by using a very short-acting medication like triazolam. However, when used as a sleeping pill, a short-acting medication can cause the person to wake up partway through the night with rebound insomnia, as the brain reacts to the rapid decrease in medication level.

Alprazolam (Xanax) and clonazepam (Klonopin) are different from the other benzodiazepines in that they *may* have mood-stabilizing properties. Clonazepam (Klonopin) is a long-acting, sedating benzodiazepine that is commonly used as an anticonvulsant and may have mood-stabilizing properties as well.

TABLE 10. *Profiles of Common Benzodiazepines*

	Half-life in Hours	Dose Range (mgs)	Speed of Onset	Addiction Potential
alprazolam (Xanax)	9–20	0.5–4	++	Higher
chlordiazepoxide (Librium)	28–100	15–100	++	Lower
clonazepam (Klonopin)	19–60	1.5–8	++	Moderate
diazepam (Valium)	30–200	2–40	++++	Higher
lorazepam (Ativan)	8–24	1–4	++	Moderate
oxazepam (Serax)	3–25	30–60	+	Lower

Key: +Slow   ++Moderate   +++Moderately fast   ++++Rapid

BUSPIRONE (BUSPAR)

This is a new class of medication that works through an entirely different mechanism of action than either the benzodiazepines or other sedative/hypnotics. It appears to be non-addictive, not habit-forming, and not subject to abuse (so far). It is the first medication to be anxiolytic (anxiety-reducing) without being sedating. It does not appear to make people more sensitive to the effects of alcohol or other sedating medications. It is not a muscle relaxant and has no anticonvulsant properties. It is also not useful in helping with alcohol or other drug withdrawal.

Buspirone does appear to have a few idiosyncrasies, which may limit its use in some people. While Valium and the other benzodiazepines appear to work almost immediately after people take their first pill, buspirone must be used regularly for up to several weeks before it is fully effective. This means it is best used as a regular medication for someone who can tolerate a delay before it begins working, rather than as a medication with rapid effects that can be taken episodically, as with Valium-type medications.

A second issue has to do with its effectiveness. Double-blind research studies have concluded that BuSpar is as effective as Valium when used by anxious subjects who have never previously used Valium. For some reason, people who have previously had much experience with Valium or Valium-type medications often feel that BuSpar is less effective. There are at least two possible interpretations to these research findings. One is that the use of Valium-type medications produces long-lasting biological changes in the brain that make BuSpar less effective, and the other is that BuSpar is not really quite as effective as Valium but that it works "well enough" for most people, unless they have already experienced the very powerful and immediate effects of Valium-type medications.

BuSpar seems particularly useful for people who are potential drug abusers and people who do not like or cannot tolerate the sedative side effects of benzodiazepines.

ANTIDEPRESSANTS AS
ANTIANXIETY MEDICATIONS

All of the antidepressants, with the exception of bupropion (Wellbutrin) are very effective antianxiety medications. Besides helping with general anxiety, as a group they are also effective for panic disorder, and much more effective than the benzodiazepines for symptoms of obsessive-compulsive disorder (OCD). Antidepressants are effective antianxiety medications even for people who are not depressed.

The antidepressants can take several weeks to work and may have more side effects than the benzodiazepines. On the other hand, they are not addictive and not subject to abuse. This makes them the medication of choice for people with a history of alcohol abuse or other addictive disorder.

SLEEPING PILLS (HYPNOTICS)

Many people who complain of insomnia are already sleeping an adequate amount but feel that they "should" be sleeping more. In some cases a person may be sleeping as much as their body needs, but they are trying to use sleep to fill up time. Other people are concerned that they cannot sleep at night but are taking naps during the day; in these cases the problem is the structure of the sleep cycle rather than a lack of sleep. Other people are depressed, and the insomnia usually improves when the depression is treated. Some people with insomnia have a specific sleep disorder, such as sleep apnea. There are specific treatments for some of these disorders, and sleeping pills may actually make things worse.

Sleep apnea is of special concern because it is fairly common and can cause major medical problems as well as depression and day time sleepiness. Most people with sleep apnea have a pattern of heavy snoring interrupted by periods of not breathing, repeated many times during the night. It is most common in people who are overweight, and the best clues often come from the snoring patterns described by the person's bed partner.

Sleeping pills are frequently necessary in the hospital because of the noise and strangeness of the hospital and general anxiety of the person. They should never be prescribed automatically, however. They should never be used in a newly admitted patient who is still intoxicated (with alcohol or some other depressant) or who still has the obvious after-effects of an overdose. They should be used with caution in older people who are likely to become confused, disoriented, or (on rare occasions) get a terrifying transient organic psychosis from sleeping pills. Finally, people with severe respiratory diseases are more apt to develop serious medical complications from the respiratory-depressant side effects of many medications, especially sleeping pills.

When I prescribe sleeping pills, I rarely give more than five pills at a time. It is sometimes nice to have a sleeping pill in the medicine closet for especially bad nights, but it is rarely necessary for anyone to use sleeping pills on a regular basis. Often, the problems caused by sleeping pills are worse than the problems caused by poor sleep.

I do *not* prescribe barbiturates, e.g., secobarbital (Seconal). They are more dangerous and more addicting. Triazolam (Halcion) used to be preferred because of its short half-life and lack of accumulation, especially in the elderly. The concern that triazolam may cause more memory impairment than other medications has led me to avoid it. Tolerance develops to all these medications (with the possible exception of zolpidem). That is, all these medications are less effective for those who take sleeping pills or tranquilizers every day.

The chronic insomnia caused by SSRI antidepressants and by ziprasidone (Geodon), the newest antipsychotic medication, presents a special problem for some people. After all of the normal approaches to sleep hygiene have been tried (decrease caffeine, exercise, stop taking naps, do not get up and smoke a cigarette, etc.), a sleeping pill can be both helpful and safe.

While all of the commonly used sleeping pills are effective, I find that the very sedating antidepressant trazodone is a safe (except for the small risk of priapism) and often effective long-term solution to the problem.

1. *Zolpidem (Ambien)* is a sleeping pill that has a similar but slightly different mechanism of action than the benzodiazepines. It is reported to be highly effective, nonaddicting, and without significant side effects. Research suggests that, unlike with the other sleeping pills, tolerance does not develop to zolpidem. This means that zolpidem continues to be effective even when taken nightly for longer periods of time. It is important to remember that the benzodiazepines were also reported to be nonaddicting when they were first introduced, and the particular abuse potential of alprazolam was not initially recognized. At the same time, zolpidem may have some real advantage over other sleeping pills. Ten mg is a typical dose for a healthy adult, and 5 mg is a typical geriatric dose.

2. *Zaleplon (Sonata)* is very similar to zolpidem. It is related to but different than a benzodiazepine and is a highly effective sleeping pill with little antianxiety action. It has an even shorter half-life than zolpidem. This means that if someone takes zolpidem and feels "hung over" the next morning, zaleplon may be a better choice. If someone takes zaleplon and wakes up in the middle of the night, than the slightly longer action of zolpidem may be a better choice.

3. *Trazodone (Desyrel)* is a sedative antidepressant that can be used as a safe and effective hypnotic, especially for the insomnia caused by SSRI-type antidepressants. A typical dose is 50–400 mg before bed. Dry mouth is a common side effect. Priaprism (prolonged, painful erection of the penis) is an uncommon but potentially dangerous side effect in men. A major advantage is that it is not addictive and is relatively safe if taken in an overdose.

4. *Temazepam (Restoril)* is a short-acting benzodiazepine that is both safe and effective. The relatively short half-life means

that the medication does not accumulate from one night to the next as does flurazepam. The usual dose is 15 mg before bedtime. It may be a bit more addictive than zolpidem or zaleplon, but there is not a lot of good data about this.

5. *Flurazepam (Dalmane)* is very similar to diazepam (Valium) with all of its side effects and advantages. It is rarely lethal in an overdose (unless taken along with alcohol), and it usually provides a comfortable night's sleep, although some people taking it report having a hangover the next morning. It is a very long acting medication, however, with a half-life (including active metabolites) of 40–250 hours. It tends to be longer in older people. This means that half of the medication can remain in the body four days after one pill is taken. If a person uses flurazepam every night, the dose from one night is added to the remaining medication from previous nights. This accumulation is a particular problem in elderly people, who can easily become confused or appear demented as the serum level of flurazepam increases. The usual dose is 15 mg before bedtime.

6. *Diphenhydramine (Benadryl)* is a sedating antihistamine that can be used as a safe, mild, sleeping medication. The biggest problem with diphenhydramine is its anticholinergic side effects (blocks on the action of acetylcholine). These include dry mouth, constipation, and blurred vision. More importantly, anticholinergic medications like diphenhydramine can also cause confusion, especially in the elderly or in people who are already taking other anticholinergic medications (including many of the antidepressants or antipsychotic medications). Diphenhydramine has already been mentioned as a treatment for muscular side effects from antipsychotic medications. The recommended dose is 50–100 mg before bed, with instructions that the person may repeat that dose in one hour. Other sedating antihistamines are also available, including hydroxyzine (Vistaril).

7. *Chloral hydrate* is an older medication that is still sometimes used in a hospital because it is inexpensive. It is well toler-

ated and effective. Unfortunately, people become habituated to chloral hydrate fairly rapidly, and after a few days it often becomes less effective. It is a more dangerous medication to overdose on than the sleeping medications now in common use. As a result, I no longer prescribe it outside of the hospital. It has a relatively short half-life, 7–10 hours, so dose accumulation is less a problem than with flurazepam. A typical dose is 500 mg before bed for older people and 1,000 mg before bed for young, healthy adults, with an additional 500 mg an hour later if the person still cannot sleep.

TABLE 11. *Profiles of Common Sleeping Medications*

Medication	Class	Half-life (hours)	Dose Range (mg)	Speed of Onset	Addiction Potential
diphenhydramine (Benadryl)	Antihistamine	1–3	25–100	++	Low
flurazepam (Dalmane)	Benzodiazepine	48–150	15–30	+++	Moderate
temazepan (Restoril)	Benzodiazepine	3–25	15–30	++	Moderate
trazodone (Desryl)	Sedating antidepressant	4–9	50–200	+++	Very low
zolpidem (Ambien)	Imidazopyridine	2–5	5–10	+++	Low
zaleplon (Sonata)	Pyrazolopyrimidine	1	5–10	++++	Low

Key: +Slow ++Moderate +++Rapid ++++Very rapid

7

Miscellaneous Medications

There are a few common types of medications that seemed important to include in this book but did not neatly fit into one of the four main categories. These are all somewhat "special purpose" medications that are a bit outside of the basic treatment of mental illness. Within this chapter, I have included six categories of miscellaneous medications:

- Antiparkinsonian medications, which are used primarily to treat the motor side effects of antipsychotic medications
- Beta-blockers, e.g., propranolol (Inderol)
- Alpha adrenergic blockers, e.g., clonidine (Catepress)
- Cognitive enhancers
- Stimulants
- Drugs to treat alcohol dependence and abuse

ANTIPARKINSONIAN MEDICATIONS

Some of the medications commonly used for Parkinson's disease are also useful in treating the Parkinsonian-like, muscle-related side effects of the antipsychotic medications. The atypical antipsychotic medications are much less likely to cause Parkinsonian side effects, and as a result the need for anticholinergic medication is much less than it used to be. Some people do get Parkinsonian or motor side effects even with atypical antipsychotics. In addition, some people continue to use traditional antipsychotic medications, either because they need a long-acting injection or because in rare cases the newer medications do not work as well.

As was already discussed, the extrapyramidal, muscle-related side effects (EPS) include dystonias (muscle spasms), tremors, akathisia (motor restlessness), and akinesia (decreased spontaneity of movements and thought).

Anticholinergics, e.g., Benztropine (Cogentin)

Most antiparkinsonian medications used in psychiatry are anticholinergic. They block acetylcholine receptors throughout the body (cholinergic refers to acetylcholine receptors, so anticholinergic refers to medications that block acetylcholine). It appears that acetylcholine and dopamine are in balance in the part of the brain that controls many involuntary muscle movements. When dopamine is blocked by an antipsychotic medication, this system becomes out-of-balance and EPS effects result. (Voluntary muscle movements are controlled by the pyramidal system. Extrapyramidal refers to the motor system outside of the pyramidal system.) One common way to treat these EPS effects is to block acetylcholine, which to some extent restores the dopamine/acetylcholine balance in this part of the brain.

Blocking acetylcholine causes problems of its own, however. While anticholinergic medications are useful for the muscle-related side effects of antipsychotic medications, they can worsen many other side effects, including dry mouth and sedation.

Side Effects. Most antiparkinsonian medications cause the same autonomic side effects as other medications with anticholinergic effects, including clozapine and the older tricyclic antidepressants. These side effects include dry mouth, blurred vision, and constipation. Less frequently, urinary retention, nasal congestion, and muscular weakness become problems. These medications can cause some kinds of glaucoma to worsen or can precipitate glaucoma in people who are already predisposed to develop it.

All these medications can cause memory and other cognitive impairments, especially in elderly people. It is important to remember that while these medications make some side effects of the antipsychotic medications better, they make other side effects worse.

Finally, these medications are nonaddictive but are sometimes abused. They produce a strange kind of "altered state" that some people find enjoyable; as a result, they have street value. In higher doses they produce a delirium where the person becomes disoriented, loses touch with reality, and sometimes becomes delusional or starts hallucinating. This delirium can be confused with psychosis. When a person on an anticholinergic medication (which can include many of the antipsychotics and antidepressants) becomes confused and out of touch with reality, it is important to determine whether the person is psychotic or delirious.

Specifics of Use. Benztropine (Cogentin) should be taken at 1–8 mg/day, often in divided doses. Many people feel that taking the medication once a day is enough, but all antiparkinsonian medications are fairly short-acting and most people will find that they "wear off" if not taken at least twice a day. I usually start with 1 mg once or twice a day, except with elderly people, who need lower doses and with whom much more caution should be taken. On prn (use only as needed) orders I usually write for 2 mg by mouth or intramuscular injection. With severe dystonias or akathisia, the person might be so uncomfortable that intramuscular or intravenous medication is best. Other commonly used anticholinergic antiparkinsonian medications include trihexyphenidyl (Artane), usual dose 2–15 mg/day; procyclidine (Kemadrin), usual dose 6–20 mg/day; and biperiden (Akineton), usual dose 2–8 mg/day.

Diphenhydramine (Benadryl)

This is a sedating antihistamine that can also be used as a sedative hypnotic (sleeping pill). It also has strong anticholinergic properties that make it useful for treating medication-induced extrapyramidal side effects. Its anticholinergic effects and mild sedation make it particularly useful for treating akathisia in some people. Its side effects are very similiar to the other anticholinergic medications.

Amantadine (Symmetrel)

Amantadine has a completely different mechanism of action than the other medications used to treat EPS effects. The antipsychotic medications all work by blocking the action of dopamine. This dopamine blockade accounts for the antipsychotics' beneficial effects as well as their EPS effects. The anticholinergic medications work by blocking the action of the neurotransmitter acetylcholine. Dopamine and acetylcholine work to balance each other in the part of the brain that controls for extrapyramidal movement. The antipsychotic medications disrupt the balance by blocking dopamine, and the anticholinergics restore the balance by blocking acetylcholine. Amantadine, on the other hand, seems to work by selectively boosting the action of the neurotransmitter dopamine. The best guess about the action of amantadine is that it boosts the action of dopamine in the part of the brain that is associated with extrapyramidal and other side effects and has minimal or no effects on dopamine in the part of the brain associated with the antipsychotic properties of the antipsychotic medications.

Amantadine has no anticholinergic side effects and many people tolerate it better than other antiparkinsonian medications. Unfortunately, amantadine is less reliable than the anticholinergic medications are, and it may lose its effectiveness over time in some people. Occasionally people discontinue amantadine immediately after starting it because they report that it makes them extremely anxious. However, this is unusual and the medication is typically well tolerated. It is now suggested that besides blocking the EPS effects of the antipsychotic medications, amantadine may also block other autonomic side effects of the antipsychotics, including weight gain and decreased libido.

The usual dose is 100 mg twice a day, which may be increased to 300 mg/day.

BETA-BLOCKERS

Beta-blockers are most commonly used to lower high blood pressure, but they have a large number of other functions. They can decrease the tremors caused by lithium, are extremely effective in performance anxiety, and may decrease rage reactions in some people.

Beta-blockers do exactly what their name says: they block the "beta" epinephrine receptors. Epinephrine is a naturally occurring chemical within the body that is released by nerve cells and the adrenal gland. It stimulates receptor sites on nerve cells, blood vessels, and other parts of the body. Receptors that are stimulated by epinephrine (or its similar first cousin, norepinephrine) are called adrenergic receptors. There are two distinct kinds of receptors called alpha-adrenergic and beta-adrenergic. Beta-blockers, e.g., propranolol (Inderal), simply block these beta receptor sites. These occur throughout the body, which partially explains why these medications are used in conditions that seem unrelated.

Indications for Use

1. *Cardiovascular uses.* Beta-blockers have traditionally been used to help control high blood pressure, treat angina, and control certain kinds of arrhythmias (irregular heartbeats). Beta-blockers are often used to treat migraine headaches, as well as to treat some more unusual conditions associated with an outpouring of epinephrine or norepinephrine.
2. *Tremors.* Benign tremors respond well to these medications. Beta-blockers in low doses are also very effective in treating the tremor that is a common side effect of lithium.
3. *Performance anxiety.* Beta-blockers are extremely effective in helping people with performance anxiety. The musician or public speaker whose anxiety begins to interfere with his or her performance often has a dramatic response to these medications, used in a very low dose. The anticipatory anxiety before the performance is still there, but the specific perfor-

mance anxiety can be decreased without any sedation or interference with cognitive or motor abilities.

4. *Anxiety with marked somatic (physical) symptoms.* Beta-blockers block some of the peripheral symptoms of anxiety. The person may still "think" anxious, but these medications can stop the pounding heart, sweaty palms, tremor, etc., that cause the anxiety to feed upon itself and get out of control. These are most useful as antianxiety agents in people who, in fact, have a lot of somatic manifestations of their anxiety.

5. *Akathisia.* Propranolol is also useful as a treatment for akathisia (the motor restlessness caused by antipsychotic medications). Even though akathisia is much less common with the new atypical antipsychotic medications, it still exists and is extremely uncomfortable.

6. *Violent outbursts.* Some research has suggested that propranolol may be useful in treating certain kinds of violent outbursts, including some of the aggressive behaviors seen in some people with development delay. It also may be useful in treating some people with schizophrenia. The dose range is moderate to high—100–2,500 mg/day. Using very high doses may be dangerous, although those dangers are somewhat unclear.

7. *"Atypical" beta-blockers: Pindolol (Viskin).* As discussed in the beginning of this book, all medications have multiple sites of action. Pindolol (Viskin), an atypical beta-blocker, not only blocks the beta norepinephrine receptor but also blocks serotonin reuptake (and therefore increases serotonin in the synapse). While most beta-blockers can potentiate depressions, pindolol may allow some antidepressants to begin to work more rapidly. Initially it was hoped that pindolol might increase how well antidepressants work as well as how fast they work, but so far this does not seem to be the case. While there have been studies that suggested that some people with treatment-resistant depressions had an improved response when pindolol was added to the antidepressant, a recent study suggests it does not help. A typical dose is 2.5

mg three times a day. It appears to be less effective with sertraline, probably because of drug-drug interactions.

Side Effects

For the most part, the beta-blockers are very safe when used in relatively low doses. They can be extremely dangerous, however, for people with asthma or chronic obstructive pulmonary disease. They can also block the clinical recognition of hypoglycemia (low blood sugar). Since people with diabetes may have serious hypoglycemic episodes, the use of beta-blockers in people with diabetes can be dangerous.

The beta-blockers can also cause or potentiate depression, especially in the higher doses used to treat high blood pressure and certain cardiac conditions. They can also cause nightmares and a sense of fatigue.

ALPHA-ADRENERGIC RECEPTOR BLOCKER: CLONIDINE (CATAPRESS)

Alpha-adrenergic receptor blockers block the alpha part of the adrenergic system. As with the beta-blockers, the most common medical use for these medications is to lower high blood pressure, but there is increasing interest in clonidine for psychiatric use.

Indications for Use

1. *Posttraumatic stress disorder.* There has been recent interest in using clonidine for posttraumatic stress disorder (PTSD). There is little controlled research, but there have been anecdotal reports and uncontrolled studies suggesting its effectiveness in the PTSD commonly seen in refugees of war-torn areas. Clonidine seems to help the hyperarousal and intrusive thoughts common to this disorder. It can be used along with an antidepressant for patients with both PTSD and depression.
2. *Drug withdrawal.* Clonidine has also been used to help manage the withdrawal symptoms associated with a number of

narcotics, from opiates to cocaine. There is relatively little good data about this use, but clonidine does seem helpful for at least some people.

Side Effects

The most common side effect is fatigue. Other side effects include dry mouth, dizziness, constipation, and skin rashes.

Specifics of Use

Clonidine is usually started at 0.1 mg once a day, and slowly increased as needed up to a maximum of 0.4–0.6 mg/day in divided doses. It is also available as a patch that lasts for seven days. It generally takes two to three days for someone to get a full serum level after first applying the patch.

STIMULANTS

Stimulants, e.g., amphetamine (Dexadrine) and methylphenidate (Ritalin), have had a somewhat checkered career in psychiatry. There are situations where stimulants are clearly useful and safe, but they have been so subject to overuse and abuse that many avoid prescribing them.

For most purposes, the various stimulants are more similar than they are different. One may be more effective than another or have slightly different side effects, but they are used for the same problems and all have more or less similar side effects.

Amphetamines

Amphetamines are used frequently with hyperactive children. Stimulants work paradoxically in children (whether hyperactive or not), helping calm them down and increase their attention spans. In normal adults, these medications do just the opposite. There is no question that amphetamines are helpful in calming hyperactive children. They help hyperactive children behave more appropriately at home and in school and enable many of these children to stay in normal classes rather than be placed in a special education program. However, there is ongoing debate about whether hyperactivity is overdiagnosed, and whether many of these children would do better with social or psychological counseling rather than pharmacological intervention.

The use of stimulants in hyperactive adults is receiving increased attention, although the research is still very scanty. Adults who have a clear history of childhood hyperactivity (which is often coupled with some history of learning disability or impulsive behavior) and who continue to have very short attention spans may be helped by stimulants.

Stimulants also have a prominent role in the treatment of resistant depressions. Most depressed people will respond much better to standard antidepressants, but a small number of depressed people who have not responded to anything else will respond very well to small amounts of amphetamine. This is indicated only in unusual situations where there is a clear biological component to the depression, when abuse seems unlikely, and when other somatic treatments have been ineffective. The use of stimulants to treat depression in the elderly has recently caught renewed attention. Elderly people often have major problems with the side effects of typical antidepressants, and stimulants may be a safe and effective alternative for some people. Amphetamines are also the medications of choice with narcolepsy.

A typical dose of amphetamine is 5–40 mg/day. Sometimes people respond well to the drug initially but later develop tolerance, so that the medication loses all effect. Within reason, the dose of the medication can be raised or another stimulant can be tried. Commonly used amphetamine preparations are: dextroamphetamine (Dexedrine), dextroamphetamine + amphetamine (Adderall), and methamphetamine (Desoxyn).

Side Effects. When they are abused, amphetamines cause a "high" or rush that some people find extremely pleasurable. Illicit amphetamines are sold as "speed" and "ice," a new form of crystalline amphetamine that is extremely pure and very potent. When used in high doses, amphetamines can produce a psychosis that resembles paranoid schizophrenia. Even a low dose of amphetamines can cause some individuals to become paranoid. When used in therapeutic doses, amphetamines and other stimulants can cause feelings of anxiety, being "wired," and agitation. Amphetamines can also cause problems with sleep, loss of appetite, increased blood pressure, and rapid or irregular pulse. They can cause tics to worsen. There is also concern that the long-term use of stimulants in children may retard normal physical growth.

Methylphenidate (Ritalin)

Methylphenidate is a stimulant that is less addicting and generally causes fewer side effects than amphetamine. It is most commonly used to treat attention deficit disorder (ADD) in both children and adults. The most common side effects are nervousness and insomnia, although nausea, diarrhea, rashes, increased blood pressure, and increased pulse have been reported. A typical dose of methyphenidate for adults is 20–40 mg/day, but some people require up to 80 mg/day. It is a short-acting medication and typically must be taken two or three times a day.

There is a long-acting form of methylphenidate (Ritalin-SR) that can be given twice a day. The dose of Ritalin-SR is supposed to be the same as regular Ritalin, but anecdotal clinical evidence suggests that a higher dose of the longer-acting preparation may be required to achieve the same effect.

Modafanil (Provigil)

Modafanil is a stimulant that has less direct dopaminergic activity than the other stimulants. This means that it should be less subject to abuse and less likely to cause psychotic symptoms. It is approved for attention deficit disorder, but initial experience suggests that it is useful for the sedative side effects of clozapine and similar medications.

COGNITIVE ENHANCERS: MEDICATIONS TO TREAT ALZHEIMER'S DISEASE

Alzheimer's disease effects many different neurotransmitter systems in the brain—acetylcholine seems to be particularly impacted. It has been found that medications that decrease or block acetylcholine tend to impair memory. All of the anticholinergic medications used to treat Parkinson's disease or Parkinsonian side effects cause some degree of memory impairment. This is worse in older people or people who already have some degree of impairment but is measurable even in younger people. All medications that increase acetylcholine activity in the brain tend to improve memory, at least in those with Alzheimer's disease. Until recently there was no way of easily and safely increasing acetylcholine in the brain, but recently a number of medications that do this have been introduced. As a group, they work by blocking acetylcholinesterase, the main enzyme that breaks apart and deactivates acetylcholine.

All are indicated for Alzheimer's disease. While these medications will not prevent or reverse the eventual deterioration seen in Alzheimer's, they can delay cognitive loss and help to maintain function. They are most effective in people with mild to moderate dementia, although recent data suggests that they can be helpful in people with more severe illness as well. *It is strongly recommended that people start on an anticholinesterase inhibitor as soon as an Alzheimer's diagnosis is made.* People started on these medications earlier in their illness have a slower downhill course and continue to have better function than people who start the medication later.

Some people respond very well to these medications, very significantly slowing the course of the illness and to some extent even reversing some of the already existing cognitive deficits. Other people have a more modest respond. While a higher dose of an anticholinesterase inhibitor can lead to more side effects, primarily nausea, a higher dose is also more likely to lead to a better response over time. If the person can tolerate the side effects, he or she is more likely to have a better response if they take the medication at the upper end of the dose range.

There is also research under way about whether these same medications will help reverse some of the cognitive impairments seen in people with schizophrenia or even reverse some of the memory problems seen in normal aging. So far there is speculation that these medications may help, but little data supports this use.

Tacrine

Tacrine was the first-known cognitive enhancer. It was effective in improving the cognitive performance of people with Alzheimer's, but it needed to be taken four times a day and was associated with serious liver problems. GI disturbance, nausea, and vomiting were common side effects. As a result, Tacrine is now used infrequently.

Donepezil (Aricept)

Donepezil was at least as effective as tacrine, while also being much safer and easier to tolerate. It was found that increasing the dose more slowly led to fewer GI side effects. Donepezil is the only anticholinesterase inhibitor currently available that can be taken just once a day. It is now started at 5 mg/day and increased over several weeks to 10 mg/day.

Galantamine (Reminyl)

Galantamine has been found to both decrease the rate of decline of memory and other cognitive functions and to improve memory in people with mild dementia. Galantamine has direct effects on nicotinic receptors, in addition to its effect on acetylcholine. This may make it more effective in improving cognitions in specific conditions, such as schizophrenia, but research on this is just beginning. It is usually started at 8 mg/day, and slowly increased to 24 mg/day.

Rivastigmine (Exalon)

Rivastigmine is short-acting, so it should be taken twice a day. It is the only medication in this group that inhibits acetylcholinesterase (Ache) and also butyrylcholinesterase (BchE). Some researchers have suggested that this dual action may lead to increased efficacy, although so far there is little data to support this idea. It is started at 1.5 mg twice a day and increased to 3–6 mg twice a day.

Side Effects. All of the newer cognitive enhancers have very similar side effects, based on their mechanism of action of increasing acetylcholine. About half of the people taking these medications experience nausea, and nausea is the most common reason that people discontinue the medication. Other side effects are rarer, and include vomiting, diarrhea, dizziness, and fatigue. These side effects can be decreased by starting the medication at a lower dose and increasing the dose slowly.

MEDICATIONS USED IN THE TREATMENT OF ALCOHOL DEPENDENCE

Disulfiram (Antabuse)

Disulfiram can be extremely useful for patients who feel that they cannot control their impulsive use of alcohol. A person will become extremely ill if he or she consumes alcohol within a few days of taking disulfiram. This means that someone who decides to drink while taking disulfiram must wait up to a week or more before actually taking the first drink. For some people, this period of enforced reflection is extremely useful.

Disulfiram has significant limitations. Many people refuse to take it or go off it to resume drinking. Some people can drink even while taking disulfiram, either because they become less ill or because they can get drunk enough to not feel the discomfort caused by the medication. A full disulfiram-alcohol reaction can be dangerous, especially in someone with other serious medical problems, particularly heart disease. Many people can get a disulfiram-alcohol reaction from cough medicine or mouthwash that contains alcohol. Disulfiram has other significant drug-drug interactions. It can increase the serum level of commonly used medications, such as phenytoin (Dilantin). Disulfiram's side effects include liver disease, rashes, fatigue, headaches, and, at times, psychosis. These side effects are dose-related and are less frequent if the dose is kept at 250 mg/day.

Naltrexone (ReVia)

Naltrexone blocks natural opiate receptors in the brain. It has been used for many years to block the effects of drugs like heroin. It is now clear that it can also decrease alcohol craving and significantly increase abstinence when it is used as part of a comprehensive alcohol treatment program. The initial research on naltrexone was for three to six months; initially it was suggested that the medication should be discontinued after six months. While there is concern about the increasing risk of liver damage with long-term use, some people are much more likely to maintain their sobriety if it is continued for a longer period of time.

Naltrexone will both decrease craving and the sense of pleasure that comes with alcohol use. As a result, even if someone relapses, he or she will be much more likely to have a drink or two and then stop instead of proceeding to a destructive out-of-control binge.

It has been suggested that naltrexone may decrease self-injuring behavior and other kinds of addictive-type behavior. There are scattered reports of using naltrexone for the self-abuse that some people with developmental delays engage in. There is also a report of using it for pathological gambling.

Naltrexone will precipitate sudden, very uncomfortable withdrawal in anyone who has recently used any opiate such as heroin or morphine. Before starting the medication, patients should be asked about opiate use and the risk of withdrawal should be explained. There is also some risk of liver damage, especially at larger doses and perhaps when used over a longer period of time. Naltrexone is usually well tolerated, but it can cause insomnia, anxiety, abdominal pain, nausea, and decreased energy in some patients. A typical dose is 50 mg/day.

8

Using Medication as a Tool for People Diagnosed with Borderline Personality Disorder

The previous sections of this book have been about medications. As I discussed, medications are tools that people can use to overcome the symptoms and disabilities caused by their mental illnesses. The relationship between the person taking the medication and the person prescribing the medication is critically important. This relationship determines whether the assessment will be accurate, whether the medication will be taken, and whether the medication is seen as a tool or just one more way that the person labeled "client" or "patient" has lost control over life. The prescriber must be technically knowledgeable about the medication but must also be skilled and interested in establishing a healing and trusting relationship. This is true throughout psychiatry and throughout medicine, but it is particularly true when working with people who have difficulty in establishing and maintaining stable relationships.

Many books have been written about people diagnosed with borderline personality disorder and more will come in the future. There are disagreements about the nature of the disorder, its cause, and certainly its treatment. One area where there is widespread agreement is that this term is applied to people who continue to have unstable relationships with others. This is in fact the core problem that leads to the diagnosis. Medications can be very effective tools for people with this diagnosis, but only if the relationship issues are attended to first. There is nothing in this section that would not apply to anyone taking medication; the issue of the relationship is most likely to interfere with the effective use of medication in this population.

I talk with many people who have a borderline diagnosis who tell me that medications do not work for them. They have been on Prozac for a week, Zoloft for two days, risperidone for three days, and Depakote for two weeks—none of them worked. They often feel frustrated by their attempts to work with prescribers. They are often both desperate for some kind of help that will help them deal with their pain and their life chaos, wishing that medication was the answer. At the same time, they are often "noncompliant," and end up using medications in ways that allow little chance of success.

A "personality disorder" is not a symptom as much as a way of living in the world that does not work well for the person. It is a pervasive, persistent, maladaptive behavior pattern that effects many areas of the person's life. We all have different ways of protecting ourselves from stress and from perceived threats. We all have bits and pieces of effective as well as maladaptive behavior. For people with a personality disorder, their ways of protecting themselves cause overwhelming and recurrent problems for themselves and for others around them.

Any label gives very incomplete information. A particular diagnosis, including that of borderline personality disorder, does not tell us anything about whether or not a person is smart, creative, generous, artistic, or all of the other attributes and strengths that are important to who we are. Diagnosis is shorthand that describes a small number of attributes that seem to fall into a pattern. Some of the criteria that go into having a diagnosis of borderline personality disorder include the following *DSM-IV* criteria:

- Avoidance of abandonment
- Unstable, intense, interpersonal relationships
- Identity disturbance
- Potentially self-damaging impulsiveness
- Recurrent suicidal or self-mutilating behavior
- Affective instability
- Chronic feelings of emptiness or boredom
- Inappropriate anger

- Transient paranoid ideation or severe dissociative symptoms

Not everyone with this diagnosis has all of these symptoms, but the overall sense is of someone who lives a life of chronic crisis and interpersonal instability. At the same time, people with a borderline diagnosis may have many skills and area of competence. They may be extremely bright and creative and may excel in work environments. Overall, however, their life is far from what they would like it to be.

I find it useful to think about the underlying problems experienced by people with borderline personality disorder. There are many different lists of "core deficits," but I think of them as the following:

1. *Affective instability.* The person switches from being depressed to being happy to being suicidal, often rapidly and without clear reason. For many people with this diagnosis, this has happened since early childhood. It probably has a large biological component and leads to a sense of not being able to trust one's own feelings since they unpredictably change.

2. *Sense of self as being damaged/defective/not good.* The vast majority of people with a borderline personality disorder have had a history of recurrent, often prolonged, sexual abuse. Others have had other kinds of profoundly invalidating experiences. Not all people with this diagnosis have had these kinds of horrific childhood experiences, and many people with sexual abuse or other invalidating experiences do not develop a borderline disorder. At the same time, the childhood experience seems relevant.

3. *Difficulty maintaining their own sense of identity/poor object constancy.* This follows from the first two problems. If you have a changing mood state, you learn you cannot trust your own feelings. If you also have recurrent abuse from someone who is supposed to protect you, you learn that you cannot trust the outside world either. It is easy to imagine how without either internal or external anchors, someone can feel defective, confused, and lost.

4. *Impulsiveness and low frustration tolerance.* Impulsiveness and problems dealing with frustration seem to follow automatically for many people with the other core deficits. Our sense of our self and our feeling of our own competency that we can cope both aid us as we cope with frustration.

Medication will not correct all of the issues that people with this disorder face, but it can provide help with specific symptoms. Medication can help with the affective lability as well as some of the anxiety, depression, and impulsiveness that are all common problems. The problem is that medications can only help part of the problem, and the person must be willing to accept and use a tool that is only partially effective.

It is important to establish a nonblaming approach to treatment. Treatment should start from the premise that the problem is caused by a lack of necessary skills that can be learned. The issue is not one of a "bad" or unmotivated person, but of someone who is unable either because of skill deficits, biological issues, or personal trauma to control their own behavior. This brief book on psychopharmacology is not even a basic primer for the treatment of people with borderline personality disorder, but some ideas about treatment are necessary to set a context in which medication can be useful. It is difficult to prescribe for a patient who is impulsive, angry, and tends to have major issues with control. Medication only has a chance of actually being taken and being effective if used within a stable clinical relationship.

ASSUMPTIONS ABOUT PEOPLE WITH BORDERLINE PERSONALITY DISORDER (BPD) AND THERAPY*

People with BPD are doing the best they can

- People with BPD want to improve.
- People with BPD need to do better, try harder, and be more motivated to change.

---

*This section is adapted from Marsha Linehan. (1993). *Cognitive-Behavioral Treatment of Borderline Personality Disorder*. New York: Guilford.

- People with BPD may not have caused all of their own problems, but they have to solve them anyway.
- The lives of suicidal, borderline individuals are unbearable as they are currently lived.
- People with BPD must learn new behaviors in all relevant contexts.
- People with BPD cannot fail in therapy.

Therapists treating people with BPD need support

- The goal is to stay in a long-term, stable relationship.
- Know the limits of your responsibility.
- Be aware of your own feelings.
- Monitor and regulate interpersonal distance.
- Be aware of "splitting"—being "right" may be less important than being part of a team.
- Be clear about the therapy contract.

Before Starting a Medication Trial

Before starting a medication trial with a person who has a borderline personality diagnosis, some basic information needs to be collected. Medication is a tool that can help someone accomplish things. This is much less likely to be useful if both the person prescribing the medication and the person given the medication are not sure what they want to accomplish.

1. What does the person prescribed the medication want?
   - What are the person's treatment goals?
   - What would "doing better" or "doing worse" mean? Be concrete and specific.
   - What commitment is the person willing and able to make?
2. What do you want?
   - What are you able to deliver? Do not promise more than you can provide.
   - What can you not tolerate? Do not agree to something that you cannot continue to support.

- What behaviors would make it difficult for you to continue the relationship?
- How far are you able to go in supporting the person?

3. Obtain a careful medication and life history.

- Assess the person's strengths. How has the person managed to survive in his or her chaotic world?
- In what areas has the person developed resiliency?
- Where does he or she get support?
- When has the person done well? What have been the person's most stable relationship, best job, and best period of function?
- Consider that problem behavior is exacerbated by treatable medical illness, a coexisting mental illness, or the sequela of trauma.
- Always consider substance abuse.

4. Review the patient's pharmacological treatment carefully and in detail.

- What has been tried? How much for how long?
- What has worked, even a little?
- What has not worked?
- What has been tried but discontinued quickly? What side effects were particularly bothersome?

Elements of a Medication Trial

1. *Develop a collaborative relationship with shared treatment goals before starting any medication.* If this basic step cannot be accomplished, it is highly unlikely that medication will be used or useful. Spend as much time as necessary to work on this, even if it takes months. A corollary of this is that the prescriber can never want a person with a borderline diagnosis to take medication more than the person themselves wants the medication. Trying too hard to "sell" or coerce medication is highly likely to lead to fights over control rather than effective treatment.

2. *Identify specific target symptoms.* If a person is now suicidal much of the time, a target symptom may be to feel less sui-

cidal. The important thing is to be concrete about what the target symptom would mean. If the person initially feels suicidal several times a day, feeling suicidal only once a day would be an improvement.

3. *Discontinue medication if target symptoms do not improve.* The hardest part of prescribing is not starting a new medication; it is stopping an old one even if it is not effective. An individual taking a medication often feels that it was doing "something," or other staff may be concerned that the person will be even worse without it. As a result it is easy for people with borderline personality disorder to end up on a list of multiple medications—none of which work very well but all potentially cause side effects.

4. *Medication decisions are never an emergency.* People with a diagnosis of borderline personality disorder often live chaotic lives of chronic crises. They may call, feeling desperate that something must be done *now*, that the medication decision cannot wait for reflection, education, and joint planning. Medications all take some time to work. If it really is a crisis, the medication will not work fast enough to help anyway. The role of medication is to help the person stabilize their life, but medication is highly unlikely to be an effective response to a crisis unless it is part of an agreed upon and carefully considered plan.

5. *Patient education is critical.* The entire approach to people with a borderline diagnosis is to help them develop new skills, new coping capacities, and new ways of dealing with the world. Having as much information as possible about medication or any other tools will help them use those tools more effectively.

6. *Get clear agreement on what medication, for how long.* I often see people who have had multiple ineffective medication trials. The person often has had significant side effects and significant difficulty tolerating those side effects for a long-enough period of time to see if the medication will do any good. I try to plan with the patient how long it will take to see if the medication will really work and to get a promise

that the patient will try to stay on the medication for that entire period of time. If the patient is unable to commit to this, I wait to start the medication trial until we trust each other enough to make that commitment.

There are different ideas for how people with borderline personality disorders should use medication but very little controlled research on this subject. Even more than in other sections of this book, I have based this section on my own experiences with relatively little guidance from research literature. The biological understanding of this disorder is still very crude and constantly changing. There are no medications for "borderline," but there are medications that are useful for the symptoms of the disorder. As a result, I use medication to target specific symptoms without worrying too much about their theory or cause. The same medications used in other areas of psychiatry are used with people with borderline disorder. If someone is depressed, I consider prescribing an antidepressant. If someone becomes disorganized under stress, I consider prescribing an antipsychotic. There are some differences in how these medications are used, and these differences can be important.

MEDICATIONS IN BORDERLINE PERSONALITY DISORDER

Mood Stabilizers

Since mood instability is part of the core problem, mood stabilizers are the cornerstone of treatment for many people with this disorder. Even people who complain of severe and even suicidal depressions often have a cyclical course to their moods, with periods of feeling relatively better interspersed with periods of feeling even worse. If the depression is treated directly with an antidepressant, there is a risk that the intensity and frequency of these mood swings can actually increase.

Commonly used mood stabilizers are all useful in people with a borderline personality disorder. My experience suggests that lithium is probably less useful; I typically start with a trial of divalproex sodium (Depakote). There is actually more research demonstrating the effectiveness of carbamazepine (Tegretal), but its side effects are often more difficult to live with and it has a bit more health risk in its use. Oxcarbazepine (Trileptel), the metabolite of carbamazepine, is safer and has fewer side effects than does oxcarbazepine, but it is unclear if it is as effective.

The dose range is much wider for people with a borderline diagnosis than when the same medications are used for people with a bipolar disorder. Some people with a bipolar disorder do very well with relatively low doses of medication that would normally be felt to be too low to be effective. On the other hand, other people need a full dose. "Starting low and going slow" is the normal procedure. By starting at a very low dose and increasing the dose much more slowly than normal, it is possible to see results at lower dose levels if they are going to occur, and side effects are decreased by the slower increase.

The goal is to even out some of the mood instability without causing too many side effects or too much emotional blunting or flattening. Careful attention to dose amount can help this process. These medications can also help to decrease impulsiveness and increase "reflective delay."

Gabapentin (Neurontin). The available research data on gabapentin suggests that it is not generally useful for people with bipolar disorder. On the other hand, there is strong anecdotal experience that it is very useful for people with rapid mood cycles or mood instability. As a result it is commonly prescribed for people with borderline disorder. As with other medications, it is not always helpful but there are individuals who have responded remarkably well to this medication. It is well tolerated with relatively few side effects for most people.

Lamotrigine (Lamactil). The other available mood stabilizers are more effective on the "up" side of mood instability. Lamotrigine is the first mood stabilizer that is effective for the "down" or depressed side of the instability. It must be started at a low dose and increased very slowly because of the risk of rash. As a result, it takes months to get up to an effective dose. While lamotrigine is not at all useful as a rapid response, it is well worth trying in someone with mood instability, where depression is a major problem.

Tiagabine (Gabitril). Tiagabine is a new anticonvulsant that might be useful as a mood stabilizer. Anecdotal reports suggest that tiagabine has been very useful in some individuals, but there is very little experience and no controlled research. It seems relatively safe and well tolerated. Some people report dizziness, fatigue, and nausea as side effects.

Topirimate (Topamax). There is little data on using topirimate in this population. Topirimate is attractive because it causes weight loss rather than weight gain, and obesity is often a frequent concern. On the other hand it has significant side effects, including cognitive problems. Some people seem to do well on topirimate with few side effects, while others find it difficult to tolerate and not particularly useful. The rapid development of glaucoma is a rare but serious side effect of topirimate. Anyone taking topirimate should see a physician immediately if they experience eye pain or changes in their vision.

Antidepressants

Traditionally, antidepressants are the medications first prescribed for people with borderline personality disorder, and virtually all of the patients whom I see with this diagnosis have already had at least one trial of an SSRI or other antidepressant. All of the newer antidepressants, including the SSRIs and the other newer medications, are useful in people with atypical depressions. Traditionally, an "atypical depression" referred to depression that included significant anxiety, increased sleep, and weight gain. People with these characteristics did not respond as well to the older tricyclic-type antidepressants. It has been suggested that the newer antidepressants are also more useful than the older tricyclic medications for people who have significant rejection sensitivity and emotional lability. All of these features are typically present in people with a borderline disorder. In addition, the newer medications are all much safer if someone overdoses on one of them, which is a considerable benefit when treating people who may be chronically suicidal and impulsive.

It is unclear if any of the various classes of the newer medications have any obvious advantages. Generally one chooses a particular medication based on side effects and special properties. For example, bupropion (Wellbutrin) is the only newer antidepressant that is not helpful in people with anxiety disorders. On the other hand, bupropion is very effective as a smoking cessation aid, and it causes no weight gain and no sexual side effects.

With the development of many newer, safer, and better tolerated antidepressants, MAO inhibitors are now rarely prescribed. MAO inhibitors can still be an important part of treatment for people who have not responded to other antidepressants. MAO inhibitors are difficult to prescribe, have many side effects, and require strict adherence to avoiding a long list of common foods. They are dangerous if someone overdoses on them, they have a significant number of dangerous drug-drug interactions, and they can be fatal for someone who uses cocaine or amphetamines while taking them. Despite their danger and inconvenience, at times they can be dramatically effective. MAO inhibitors can only be used with someone who has been very well educated on both the risks and benefits of the medication, and who can follow all of the required restrictions.

People with borderline personality disorder often seem much more sensitive to side effects. There is also concern about antidepressants increasing a person's already-unstable emotional instability. For all of these reasons, I would suggest starting these medications at somewhat less than normal doses and increasing them a bit more slowly than one would with someone who has a more straightforward form of depression.

It is very important to develop and reinforce collaboration with the person about the use of the medication before starting it. The target symptoms should be clearly laid out, along with the likely timeframe that it will take the person to know whether or not it is going to work. Do not start a medication that is likely to be stopped in a few days or when the person is unlikely to agree to an increased and more effective dose.

Switching Antidepressants. Very often, the first and the second medications do not work, and then the third medication turns out to be very useful. People often respond to one of the antidepressants but not another. There is no way to predict this response, which means that a trial and error process is sometimes required.

Antipsychotics

Antipsychotic medications, often in very low doses, are often very useful in helping people with a borderline diagnosis help organize their thoughts. The atypical antipsychotic medications are better tolerated and may be more effective than the older medications. The atypical antipsychotic medications are much less likely to cause EPS effects and are much less likely to cause tardive dyskinesia. Finally, they appear to be better as mood stabilizers than the older antipsychotic medications.

Indications for Use. Many people with borderline disorder go through periods of severe anxiety. Often they become disorganized during these periods, with trouble concentrating and focusing. This anxiety often feels different than normal anxiety and is accompanied by significant distress. At times, people can develop mini-psychotic episodes, with some short-lived psychotic symptoms.

The antipsychotic medications can help with this anxiety. They can help people organize their thinking and feel less scattered. While there are some risks and side effects from the atypical antipsychotic medications, they are not addictive and not generally abused. They are also relatively safe if they are taken in an overdose.

Specifics of Use. Almost always, very low doses of antipsychotic medication are both effective and well tolerated. Doses that would be ineffective in people with schizophrenia are often very useful in people with borderline disorder. Often higher, more normal doses of these medications are less useful. Higher doses often seem less effective, and they produce more side effects. In particular, people with borderline disorder often feel "blunted" if the dose of the medication is raised past a very low level.

People with borderline disorder can take the antipsychotic medications only when needed, rather than in the same dose every day. This is very different than the way people with schizophrenia use these same medications. For some people, the antipsychotic medications can be a tool to help them cope with stress. They can help people to function without feeling so overwhelmed by everyday tasks. Again, they do not work for everyone with a borderline disorder, but they may be worth trying if anxiety and disorganization are significant problems.

In rarer situations, the atypical antipsychotic medications can also be used as primary mood stabilizers for people who have not responded to other mood stabilizers. Clozapine in particular, despite all of its risks and side effects, can be effective even when other mood stabilizers have not helped.

Choosing a Specific Antipsychotic Medication. All of the antipsychotic medications are helpful. Each has advantages and disadvantages, and it is often worth trying a second or third medication if the first one does not work as hoped.

Quetiapine is least likely to cause EPS effects. Its mild sedation often helps the person sleep, and it is generally very well tolerated. It is often used over a wide dose range, from 25 mg up to several hundred mg.

Ziprasidone is the newest antipsychotic. It often allows people to feel energized, and it is the only currently available antipsychotic that does not cause weight gain. It is well tolerated with few side effects. It sometimes causes agitation and sleep problems, however, which are significant problems for some people.

Olanzapine is very effective, mildly sedating, and generally well tolerated. In the low dose range used by people with borderline personality disorder, EPS effects are rarely a problem. It can cause significant weight gain and some increased risk of diabetes if used consistently.

Risperidone is well tolerated when used at the 1–2 mg dose range often prescribed for people with a borderline disorder. It is calming without being very sedating. Even at this dose, risperidone can cause motor restlessness and can cause prolactin elevation.

Clozapine has more side effects and more health risk than any of the other antipsychotic medications. In very rare situations, it may be worth trying as a mood stabilizer when no other medications have been effective.

Benzodiazepines

Addictive medications should be used rarely and with significant caution for people who have a history of other addictions. Given the high rate of substance abuse among people with borderline disorder and their tendency towards extremes and impulsiveness, benzodiazepines should be used only rarely and cautiously. Too often, using benzodiazepines to treat the anxiety that frequently accompanies borderline personality disorder ends up causing addiction, disinhibition, and further destabilization. In particular, benzodiazepines should almost never be used in people who already abuse alcohol or other drugs, no matter how much they request them or complain of anxiety.

If benzodiazepines are used, there should be very clear target symptoms and the amount of medication prescribed should be carefully monitored. If the person's behavior becomes more out of control, the benzodiazepines should be stopped.

Medications for Alcohol Abuse

Alcohol abuse is common in people with borderline disorder. Active treatment of alcohol and other substance abuse is an extremely important part of an overall treatment approach.

Antabuse is probably underused. It can help people who want to stop drinking but have problems controlling their impulsive use of alcohol. Someone taking antabuse has to decide several days ahead of time to drink, rather than deciding to use alcohol impulsively. On the other hand, someone who is impulsive and self-destructive can drink while taking antabuse as another form of self-abuse. Antabuse should only be prescribed for people who feel it would be helpful, and who feel that they could control any impulsive desire to drink while taking the medication.

Naltrexone decreases the craving for alcohol. This can make it easier for motivated people to stop drinking, especially if combined with an active alcohol treatment program. It has been suggested that it might help decrease some of the impulsive cutting and other destructive behaviors of borderline patients, but later research has not shown naltrexone to be effective for this.

Bibliography

Given the rate of change, a newer reference will be more up to date and therefore better than one published a few years ago. I would not buy a general psychopharmacology reference more than two or three years old. I have included some references that are now somewhat out of date but may become available in new editions.

GENERAL REFERENCES FOR NONPHYSICIANS

Gitlin, M. J. (1996). *The psychotherapist's guide to psychopharmacology* (2nd ed.). New York: Free Press.
This book is designed for the nonphysician and is very readable. It includes a lot of clinical wisdom and technical information about medication, and provides a good overview of biological psychiatry, theory, and pharmacology. It is somewhat less useful as a rapid reference book. Although on the edge of being out of date, it is still a useful overview. If a new edition were published it would be highly recommended.

Gorman, J. M. (1998). *The essential guide to psychiatric drugs* (3rd ed.). New York: St. Martin's Press.
This excellent book for clients, families, and nonmedical professionals is very readable and very well organized. It can serve as a detailed reference as questions arise. It contains much more information on more medications than other client-oriented psychopharmacology books.

Preston, J. D., O'Neal, J. H., & Talaga, M. C. (2002) *Handbook of clinical psychopharmacology for therapists* (3rd ed.). Oakland, CA: New Harbinger Publications.

Weiden, P. J., Scheifler, P. L., Diamond, R. J., Ross, R. (1999). *Switching antipsychotic medications: A guide for consumers and families.* Arlington, VA: National Alliance for the Mentally Ill.
This guide provides up-to-date information on the new atypical antipsychotic medications, with an emphasis on how to start one of the new medications and how to switch from a traditional antipsychotic to one of the new medications. It includes general information about how to most effectively use medications, as well as technical information about each of the atypical antipsychotics.

GENERAL PSYCHOPHARMACOLOGY TEXTS

Gelenberg, A. J., & Bassuk, E. L. (1997). *The practitioner's guide to psychoactive drugs* (4th ed.). New York: Plenum.
An excellent general handbook. This is on the edge of being out of date, but if a new edition were published it would be highly recommended.

Janicak, P. G., David, J. M., Preskorn, S. H., & Ayd, F. J. (2001). *Principles and practice of psychopharmacology* (3rd ed.). Philadelphia, PA: Lippincott Williams & Wilkins
This is a definitive textbook, better referenced than the second edition, with more research support. It is an excellent reference book.

Schatzberg, A. F. & Nemeroff C. B. (2001). *Essentials of clinical psychopharmacology* (4th ed.). Washington, DC: American Psychiatric Press.
A very good book, up-to-date and complete. This is more than a handbook, but less than a fully referenced textbook.

Schatzberg, A. F. & Nemeroff, C. B. (1998). *Textbook of psychopharmacology* (2nd ed.). American Psychiatric Press.
This book is now several years old, but it is still one of the definitive reference texts in psychopharmacology. It is not intended for light reading.

Werry, J. S., & Aman, M. G. (1999). *Practitioner's guide to psychoactive drugs for children and adolescents* (2nd ed.). New York: Plenum.
A very readable general overview of psychopharmacology for children and adolescents.

SPECIALIZED REFERENCE BOOKS

Bezchlibnyk-Butler, K. Z., & Jeffries, J. J. (2001). *Clinical handbook of psychotropic drugs* (11th ed.). Kirkland, WA: Hogrefe & Huber.

Drug facts and comparisons (2002). St. Louis, MO: Facts and Comparisons.
This is a compendium of all prescribed medications with indications and side effects, including very useful summary tables. It covers the same material as the *PDR*, but is much more readable. Unfortunately, it is also much more expensive than the *PDR*.

Physicians' desk reference (PDR) (56th ed.). (2002). Montvale, NJ: Thomson Medical Economics.
This book lists every prescription medication marketed in the United States, along with indications, approved dose ranges, and side effects. It has indexes for medications by trade name, generic name, and drug category. Unfortunately, it is difficult to interpret information in this book; for example, it lists every reported side effect without giving information about which side effects are common and which are not, which are serious and which are trivial. *Drug Facts and Comparisons* covers similar information in a more user-friendly format (see above), but the *PDR* is more readily available.

Stahl, S. M. (2000). *Essential psychopharmacology* (2nd ed.). New York: Cambridge University Press.
This is an excellent, very readable book on neurotransmitters, receptors, and the basic science of how medications work. It is not useful as a clinical guide, but would be highly recommended for someone who wants a more theoretical understanding of psychopharmacology.

Julien, R. M. (2000). *A primer of drug action* (9th ed.). New York: Woth Publishers.
This is an excellent, very readable overview of how medications work, how the brain is organized, and how receptors work. It includes

a very useful section on the mechanism of drugs of abuse, including marijuana, hallucinogens and anabolic steroids. Although it is somewhat technical and is not useful as a clinical guide, it is highly recommended for a more theoretical understanding of drug action.

USEFUL BOOKS, EVEN IF NOT ABOUT PSYCHOPHARMACOLOGY

Diagnostic and statistical manual of mental disorders (4th ed., text revision [DSM-IV-TR]). (2000). Washington, DC: American Psychiatric Association Press.

This is the current diagnostic manual being used in the United States. The smaller *Quick Reference Guide* includes all of the diagnosis and definitions, but not the background material.

Fadiman, A. (1997). *The spirit catches you and you fall down*. New York: Farrar, Straus and Giroux.

Officially this book has nothing to do with psychopharmacology, but it is required reading for all medical students who take an elective with me. On the surface it is about the conflict between a very well-meaning set of physicians, and a very loving Hmong family dealing with a daughter with severe epilepsy. It is really about how our own values and beliefs color everything we do. If you are part of a struggle over whether medication is needed or whether someone has a mental illness, then you too should read this book. It is the most important book that I have read over the past several years.

Hyman, S. E., & Tesar, G. E. (Eds.). (1994). *Manual of psychiatric emergencies* (3rd ed.). Boston: Little, Brown.

This is a guide for emergency psychiatry, but it is still very useful and has a lot of practical information about medications. *I highly recommend this book for crisis intervention and emergency psychiatry.* The psychopharmacology may be a bit out of date, but it is still the best book I know about emergency psychiatry.

Linehan, M. M. (1993). *Cognitive-behavioral treatment of borderline personality disorder*. New York: Guilford.

This continues to be the definitive book in the practical treatment of people with this diagnosis. It is practical, thoughtful, and respectful of the struggles that people are experiencing.

SELF-HELP BOOKS

Craske, M. G. & Barlow, D. H. (2000). *Mastery of your anxiety and panic: Therapist guide* (3rd ed.). San Diego, CA: Academic Press.
This is one of the standard self-help books that we give to people who come into our clinic with complaints of anxiety and panic. It is practical and very user friendly

Beckfield, D. F. (1998). *Master your panic and take back your life* (2nd ed.). Atascadero, CA: Impact Publishers.
This is an excellent, practical, and highly readable self-help book for dealing with panic disorder.

Greenberger, D. & Padesky, C. A. (1995). *Mind over mood*. New York: Guilford.
This self-help and clinician-training manual for dealing with depression is based on the principles of cognitive behavioral therapy initially developed by Aaron Beck. There are many self-help books for depression, and there may be others may as good as this one, but this is the one that I know and use. I regularly suggest to almost all of the clients I see with depression, and their families, read this book.

Hauri, P., Jarman, M., & Linde, S. (2001). *No more sleepless nights*. New York: John Wiley.
This book, along with its companion workbook, are excellent self-help books for people with insomnia.

Marshal, J. (1995). *Social phobia: From shyness to stage fright*. New York: Basic Books.
Social phobia is very common and frequently not diagnosed. While there are now several excellent self-help books about social phobia, this is the one I know best and recommend most often.

NEWSLETTERS

There are a number of psychopharmacology newsletters. These survey the recent literature and provide brief, practical, and up-to-date overviews of current research. They provide an easy way to stay current with the latest developments. They are all a bit different, and all are excellent. They are designed for physicians and others who are knowledgeable about psychopharmacology.

Gelenberg, A. (Ed.). *Biological therapies in psychiatry.* Tucson, AZ: Gelenberg Consulting and Publishing. Available at *www.btpnews.com*

Sakland, R. *The Brown University psychopharmacology update.* Providence, RI: Manisses Communications Group. Available at *www.manisses.com*

Ayd, F. *International drug therapy newsletter.* Philadelphia, PA: Lippincott Williams and Wilkins. Available at *www.lww.com*
This is more expensive than the other two, but all are of very high quality.

COMPUTER-BASED PROGRAMS

Medical Letter is a good, inexpensive, computer-based program for drug-drug interactions. Available at www.medletter.com

Epocrates is a program for a Palm PDA that gives basic information about every medication in the PDR. It is free and is available at www.epocrates.com

WEB SITES

www.dr-bob.org/tips/
My favorite psychopharmacology Web site is the Psychopharmacology Tips page, which is an indexed archive of the psychopharmacology discussion group. It provides information about current innovative uses of medications, recognition and treatment of side effects, and is a repository of cutting-edge information. It is based on the contributors' clinical experience, not on research, and it must be used with this in mind. It also has links to a variety of other useful pages.

www.mentalhealth.com
A Web page of general mental health information, including a pointer to a pharmacology page that includes basic information about almost every prescription medication available in the United States.

www.fda.gov/medwatch

At this site, you can search for FDA warnings about medications via a simple search engine at the Web site. You can also go into the FDA Web page to look at the data presented for new medication approvals, but this information is not well indexed and is often difficult to find.

www.nami.org

This is the Web page for the National Alliance for the Mentally Ill. It is not really a psychopharmacology site, but it is still a useful reference. Every professional, family member, and consumer who is dealing with serious mental illness should know about NAMI.

www.samhsa.gov

This is a Web site, from the Substance Abuse and Mental Health Services Administration (SAMHSA), contains a lot of good general information about statistics, grants, and government initiatives, but not much about medications.

www.mentalhealth.org

This is the knowledge exchange Web site of the Center for Mental Health Services. It includes links to many other Web sites, and allows access to all of the Surgeon General's Reports as well as to the searchable link, "Mental Health Resources on the Internet."

Drug Identification by Brand Name

Brand Name	Generic Name	Chief Action
Akineton	biperiden	Antiparkinsonian, anticholinergic
Ambiem	zolpidem	Sleeping pill
Amytal	amobarbital	Sleeping pill, barbiturate
Anafranil	clomipramine	Tricyclic antidepressant—used with OCD
Antabuse	disulfiram	Anti-alcohol
Aricept	donepezil	
Artane	trihexphenidyl	Antiparkinsonian, anticholinergic
Asendin	amoxapine	Tricyclic antidepressant
Atarax	hydroxyzine	Sedating antihistamine
Ativan	lorazepam	Antianxiety, benzodiazepine
Atropine Sulfate	atropine	Anticholinergic
Benadryl	diphenhydramine	Sedating antihistamine
BuSpar	buspirone	Antianxiety
Butisol	butabarbital	Antianxiety, barbiturate
Catapres	clonidine	Alpha adrenergic agonist
Celexa	citalopram	
Clozaril	clozapine	Atypical antipsychotic
Cogentin	benztropine	Antiparkinsonian, anticholinergic
Cylert	pemoline	Stimulant
Dalmane	flurazepam	Sleeping pill, benzodiazepine
Depakene	valproic acid	Anticonvulsant, mood stabilizer
Depakote	divalproex	Anticonvulsant, mood stabilizer
Desyrel	trazodone	Sedating antidepressant
Dexedrine	dextroamphetamine	Stimulant
Doral	quazepam	Sleeping pill
Doriden	glutethimide	Sleeping pill (no longer used)
Effexor	venlafaxine	New generation antidepressant

(continued)

Brand Name	Generic Name	Chief Action
Elavil	amitriptyline	Tricyclic antidepressant
Eldepryl	selegiline	MAOI used for Parkinson's disease
Eminyl	galantamine	
Equanil	meprobamate	Antianxiety (older medication)
Eskalith	lithium	Mood stabilizer
Exalon	rivastigmine	
Fastin	phentermine	Appetite suppressant
Gabitril	tiagamine	
Geodon	ziprasidone	Atypical antipsychotic
Halcion	triazolam	Sleeping pill, benzodiazepine
Haldol	haloperidol	Antipsychotic
Inapsine	droperidol	Antipsychotic (used in anesthesia)
Inderal	propranolol	Beta blocker
Janimine	imipramine	Tricyclic antidepressant
Kemadrin	procyclidine	Antiparkinson, anticholinergic
Klonopin	clonazepam	Antianxiety, benzodiazepine
Lamictil	lamotrigine	Anticonvulsant, mood stabilizer
Lamictil	lamotrigine	
Larodopa	levodopa	Dopamine booster used for Parkinson's disease
Librium	chlordiazepoxide	Antianxiety, benzodiazepine
Lithane	lithium	Mood stabilizer
Lithobid	lithium	Mood stabilizer
Loxitane	loxapine	Antipsychotic
Ludiomil	maprotiline	Antidepressant
Luvox	fluvoxamine	SSRI antidepressant
Marplan	isocarboxazid	MAOI antidepressant (no longer marketed)
Mellaril	thioridazine	Antipsychotic
Miltown	meprobamate	Antianxiety (older medication)
Moban	molindone	Antipsychotic
Narcan	naloxone	Narcotic antagonist
Nardil	phenelzine	MAOI antidepressant
Navane	thiothixene	Antipsychotic
Neurotin	gabapentin	Anticonvulsant, mood stabilizer
Noctec	chloral hydrate	Sleeping pill
Norpramin	desipramine	Tricyclic antidepressant
Orap	pimozide	Antipsychotic
Pamelor	nortriptyline	Tricyclic antidepressant
Paral	paraldehyde	Sleeping pill
Parlodel	bromocriptine	Dopamine agonist used for side effects
Parnate	tranylcypromine	MAOI antidepressant
Paxil	paroxetine	SSRI antidepressant

Brand Name	Generic Name	Chief Action
Placidyl	ethchlorvynol	Sleeping pill
Pondimin	fenfluramine	Appetite suppressant
Prolixin	fluphenazine	Antipsychotic
ProSom	estazolam	Sleeping pill
Prozac	fluoxetine	SSRI antidepressant
Remeron	mirtazepine	New generation antidepressant
Restoril	temazepam	Sleeping pill, benzodiazepine
ReVia	naltrexone	Narcotic antagonist
Risperdal	risperidone	Atypical antipsychotic
Risperidone Consta	risperidone micro-sphere injectable	
Ritalin	methylphenidate	Stimulant
Seconal	secobarbital	Sleeping pill, barbiturate (dangerous)
Serax	oxazepam	Antianxiety, benzodiazepine
Serentil	mesoridazine	Antipsychotic
Seroquel	quetiapine	Atypical antipsychotic
Serzone	nefazodone	New generation antidepressant
Sinemet	carbidopa-levodopa	Dopamine booster for Parkinson's disease
Sinequan	doxepine	Tricyclic antidepressant
Sonata	zaleplon	
Stelazine	trifluoperazine	Antipsychotic
Surmontil	trimipramine	Tricyclic antidepressant
Symmetrel	amantadine	Antiparkinson
Tegretol	carbamazepine	Mood stabilizer, anticonvulsant
Thorazine	chlorpromazine	Antipsychotic
Tofranil	imipramine	Tricyclic antidepressant
Topamax	topirimate	
Tranxene	clorazepate	Antianxiety, benzodiazepine
Trilafon	perphenazine	Antipsychotic
Valium	diazepam	Antianxiety, benzodiazepine
Vistaril	hydroxyzine	Sedating antihistamine
Vivactil	protriptyline	Tricyclic antidepressant
Wellbutrin	buproprion	New generation antidepressant
Xanax	alprazolam	Antianxiety, benzodiazepine
Zyprexa	olanzapine	Atypical antipsychotic

Drug Identification
by Generic Name

Generic Name	Brand Name	Chief Action
alprazolam	Xanax	Antianxiety
amantadine	Symmetrel	Antiparkinson
amitriptyline	Elavil	Tricyclic antidepressant
amobarbital	Amytal	Sleeping pill, barbiturate
amoxapine	Asendin	Tricyclic antidepressant
atropine	Atropine Sulfate	Anticholinergic
benztropine	Cogentin	Antiparkinson, anticholinergic
biperiden	Akineton	Antiparkinson, anticholingeric
bromocriptine	Parlodel	Dopamine agonist used for side effects
buproprion	Wellbutrin	New generation antidepressant
buspirone	BuSpar	Antianxiety
butabarbital	Butisol	Antianxiety, barbiturate
carbamazepine	Tegretol	Mood stabilizer, anticonvulsant
carbidopa-levodopa	Sinemet	Dopamine booster used for Parkinson's disease
chloral hydrate	Noctec	Sleeping pill
chlordiazepoxide	Librium	Antianxiety, benzodiazepine
chlorpromazine	Thorazine	Antipsychotic
citalopram	Celexa	
clomipramine	Anafranil	Tricyclic antidepressant—used with OCD
clonazepam	Klonopin	Antianxiety, benzodiazepine
clonidine	Catapres	Alpha adrenergic agonist
clorazepate	Tranxene	Antianxiety, benzodiazepine
clozapine	Clozaril	Atypical antipsychotic
desipramine	Norpramin	Tricyclic antidepressant

(continued)

Generic Name	Brand Name	Chief Action
dextroamphe-tamine	Dexedrine	Stimulant
diazepam	Valium	Antianxiety, benzodiazepine
diphenhydramine	Benadryl	Sedating antihistamine
disulfiram	Antabuse	Anti-alcohol
divalproex	Depakote	Anticonvulsant, mood stabilizer
donepezil	Aricept	
doxepine	Sinequan	Tricyclic antidepressant
droperidol	Inapsine	Antipsychotic (used in anesthesia)
estazolam	ProSom	Sleeping pill
ethchlorvynol	Placidyl	Sleeping pill
fenfluramine	Pondimin	Appetite supressant
fluoxetine	Prozac	SSRI antidepressant
fluphenazine	Prolixin	Antipsychotic
flurazepam	Dalmane	Sleeping pill, benzodiazepine
fluvoxamine	Luvox	SSRI antidepressant
gabapentin	Neurotin	Anticonvulsant, mood stabilizer
galantamine	Eminyl	
glutethimide	Doriden	Sleeping pill (no longer used)
haloperidol	Haldol	Antipsychotic
hydroxyzine	Atarax, Vistaril	Sedating antihistamine
imipramine	Tofranil, Janimine	Tricyclic antidepressant
isocarboxazid	Marplan	MAOI antidepressant (no longer marketed)
lamotrigine	Lamictil	Anticonvulsant, mood stabilizer
levodopa	Larodopa	Dopamine booster used for Parkinson's disease
lithium	Eskalith, Lithane, Lithobid	Mood stabilizer
lorazepam	Ativan	Antianxiety, benzodiazepine
loxapine	Loxitane	Antipsychotic
maprotiline	Ludiomil	Antidepressant
meprobamate	Miltown, Equanil	Antianxiety (older medication)
mesoridazine	Serentil	Antipsychotic
methylphenidate	Ritalin	Stimulant
mirtazepine	Remeron	New generation antidepressant
molindone	Moban	Antipsychotic
naloxone	Narcan	Narcotic antagonist
naltrexone	ReVia	Narcotic antagonist
nefazodone	Serzone	New generation antidepressant
nortriptyline	Pamelor	Tricyclic antidepressant
olanzapine	Zyprexa	Atypical antipsychotic
oxazepam	Serax	Antianxiety, benzodiazepine

Generic Name	Brand Name	Chief Action
paraldehyde	Paral	Sleeping pill
paroxetine	Paxil	SSRI antidepressant
pemoline	Cylert	Stimulant
perphenazine	Trilafon	Antipsychotic
phenelzine	Nardil	MAOI antidepressant
phentermine	Fastin	Appetite suppressant
pimozide	Orap	Antipsychotic
procyclidine	Kemadrin	Antiparkinson, anticholinergic
propranolol	Inderal	Beta blocker
protriptyline	Vivactil	Tricyclic antidepressant
quazepam	Doral	Sleeping pill
quetiapine	Seroquel	Atypical antipsychotic
risperidone	Risperdal	Atypical antipsychotic
risperidone micro-sphere injectable	Risperidone Consta	
rivastigmine	Exalon	
secobarbital	Seconal	Sleeping pill, barbiturate (dangerous)
selegiline	Eldepryl	MAOI used for Parkinson's disease
temazepam	Restoril	Sleeping pill, benzodiazepine
thioridazine	Mellaril	Antipsychotic
thiothixene	Navane	Antipsychotic
tiagamine	Gabitril	
topirimate	Topamax	
tranylcypromine	Parnate	MAOI antidepressant
trazodone	Desyrel	Sedating antidepressant
triazolam	Halcion	Sleeping pill, benzodiazepine
trifluoperazine	Stelazine	Antipsychotic
trihexyphenidyl	Artane	Antiparkinson, anticholinergic
trimipramine	Surmontil	Tricyclic antidepressant
valproic	Depakene	Anticonvulsant, mood stabilizer
venlafaxine	Effexor	New generation antidepressant
zaleplon	Sonata	
ziprasidone	Geodon	Atypical antipsychotic
zolpidem	Ambiem	Sleeping pill

Index